The Technique of Child Psychoanalysis

Discussions with Anna Freud

The Technique of
Child Psychoanalysis

Discussions with
Anna Freud

Joseph Sandler

Hansi Kennedy

Robert L. Tyson

HARVARD UNIVERSITY PRESS Cambridge, Massachusetts

To Anna Freud

with affection and appreciation

Copyright © 1980 by Joseph Sandler
All rights reserved
Printed in the United States of America

10 9 8 7 6 5 4 3 2

Library of Congress Cataloging in Publication Data

Sandler, Joseph.
    The technique of child psychoanalysis.

    1. Child analysis. 2. Freud, Anna, 1895–
3. Hampstead Child-Therapy Clinic, London. I. Kennedy, Hansi, joint author. II. Tyson, Robert L.,
joint author. III. Freud, Anna, 1895– IV. Title.
RJ504.2.S26   618.92'89'17   80-14052
ISBN 0-674-87100-6 (cloth)
ISBN 0-674-87101-4 (paper)

Preface

by Anna Freud

That children are more difficult to treat analytically than adults should not be a surprise to anybody. Expectations in a more optimistic direction were perhaps aroused by the early finding that children's dreams are easier to interpret than those of their seniors, with the dream distortion less elaborate and the latent dream-wish more open to view. Nevertheless, this small bonus counts little when weighed against a host of disadvantages, such as the child's diminished insight and fluctuating treatment alliance, his increased intolerance for unpleasure and anxiety, his inability or unwillingness to embark on free association, his preference for action rather than verbalization, his disinclination to bear frustration in the transference relationship, and the unavoidable intrusion of parents. It is no easy matter under these circumstances to fashion a technique which complies with the main demands of classical psychoanalysis: to interpret resistance and transference phenomena; to undo repressions and regressions and to substitute sophisticated, adaptive measures for primitive, pathogenic mechanisms of defense; and generally to strengthen the ego functions and widen the area in the mind over which the ego can exert control.

So far, the various child analytic centers have come up with their own solutions of these difficulties, varying widely with regard to the materials offered to the child as a substitute for verbal communication, the depth of interpretation aimed at, the amount of permitted gratification or implied frustration of wishes, and the inclusion or exclusion of the parents. Moreover, not infrequently it is left to the individual child analyst's ingenuity to devise ways and means for countering the patient's unwillingness or refractoriness in joining forces with the therapeutic effort.

In harmony with such earlier attempts, this publication offers the essence of a series of discussions on psychoanalytic technique as practiced at the Hampstead Clinic, focused on the most significant points of contact with the child. Although the participants were unable to arrive at a complete consensus, the book gives valuable help, hints, and suggestions to the learner in child psychoanalysis and child psychotherapy, as well as providing material for comparison and consideration by more experienced colleagues in the field.

Acknowledgments

This book owes a great deal to the staff members and students at the Hampstead Clinic, who gave of their time and effort to index their cases and to participate in the discussions on child psychoanalytic technique reported here. The project was funded by the Foundation for Research in Psychoanalysis, Beverly Hills, California, and we owe a debt of gratitude to Lita Hazen and Ralph R. Greenson, who enthusiastically sponsored the work. Besides the three authors and Anna Freud, participants in the discussions included Agi Bene-Moses, Maria Berger, Marion Burgner, Dorothy Burlingham, Rose Edgcumbe, Liselotte Frankl, Ilse Hellman, Alex Holder, Elizabeth Holder, Anne Hurry, Sheila Mason, Lily Neurath, Jack Novick, Sara Rosenfeld, Marjorie Sprince, Ruth Thomas, and Clifford Yorke. We are extremely indebted to Anna Freud—for her participation in the project, for her encouragement and support, and for permission to use her comments in the text of this book.

We also thank Doreen Ross, who typed many versions of the manuscript; Audrey Gavshon, who read some of the preliminary material and offered suggestions; Trudy McGuinness and Dorothy Unwin, who worked diligently to put the final manuscript in order; and Anne-Marie Sandler and Phyllis Tyson, who made valuable comments on the manuscript and offered persistent support and encouragement over the years this book was in preparation. We are indebted and grateful to Virginia LaPlante, our editor, for all her help and encouragement in guiding this work toward publication and for painstakingly undertaking the task of editing what was originally a most difficult text.

The Hampstead Clinic has, at various times, received financial support from The American Philanthropic Foundation, Philadelphia;

Gustave M. Berne Foundation, New York; Lionel Blitsten Memorial, Chicago; G. G. Bunzl Fund, London; H. Daroff Foundation, New York; The Division Fund, Chicago; Field Foundation, New York; Ford Foundation, New York; The Foundation for Research in Psychoanalysis, Beverly Hills, Calif.; Foundation for Research in Psychiatry, New Haven, Conn.; Freud Centenary Fund, London; Grant Foundation Inc., New York; The Estate of Flora Haas, New York; Lita Hazen Charitable Fund, Philadelphia; A. and M. Lasker Foundation, New York; Leslie Foundation, Chicago; Andrew Mellon Foundation, later Paul Mellon, Pittsburgh; Walter E. Meyer Research Institute of Law, New Haven, Conn.; National Institute of Mental Health, Bethesda, Md.; New-Land Foundation, New York; Psychoanalytic Research and Development Fund, New York; William Rosenwald Family Fund, New York; William Sachs Foundation, New York; J. and M. Schneider Foundation, New York; Philip M. Stern Foundation, Washington, D.C.; W. Clement and Jessie V. Stone Foundation, Chicago; Taconic Foundation, New York; The Wolfson Foundation, London; and a number of private donors.

J.S., H.K., and R.L.T.

Contents

Introduction   1

Part One: The Framework of Treatment

1   Scheduling and Attendance   7
2   Interruptions   17
3   Change of Therapist   26
4   Change of Setting   35

Part Two: The Therapeutic Relationship

5   Treatment Alliance   45
6   Resistance   57
7   Fantasies and Expectations   62
8   Insight and Self-Observation   67
9   Reaction to Interpretations   74
10 Transference   78
11 Other Uses of the Therapist   105

Part Three: The Child's Modes of Expression

12 Bringing in Material   117
13 Acting Out   137
14 Coming and Going   144

Part Four: Interpretation and Intervention

15 Introducing Treatment   153
16 Clarification and Confrontation   158
17 Aids to Interpretation   164
18 Significant Interpretations   170
19 Selection and Timing   175
20 Working Through   182
21 Restrictions   187
22 Physical Contact and Gratification   192
23 Modifications of Technique   199
24 Extra-Analytic Contact   209
25 Termination of Treatment   241

Part Five: The Outcome of Treatment

26 Aims of Treatment   251
27 Assessment and Follow-up   257

    Case Index   269
    General Index   270

Introduction

There is no primer of psychoanalytic technique for the treatment of adults or children. By its very nature psychoanalytic technique defies being frozen into a work of that sort. The technique of psychoanalysis is the product of a vast set of influences acting on the therapist, including his own personal psychoanalysis, his relationships with teachers and supervisors, and the range of patients to whom he is exposed during his formative years as a psychoanalyst. Last, but by no means least, is the influence of the therapist's own psychoanalytic milieu, its history and theoretical framework.

This book describes the essential features of the treatment situation in one particular psychoanalytic milieu, the Hampstead Child-Therapy Clinic in London. The Hampstead Clinic was founded by Anna Freud as a direct descendant of the Hampstead Nurseries of the Second World War. It began with the creation of a child psychoanalytic training course in 1947, and five years later, after the acquisition of a suitable building, the clinic was formally opened. Since that time it has developed into a center of training, psychoanalytic child therapy, and research in the areas of normal and pathological child development (Hansi Kennedy, "The Hampstead Centre for the Psychoanalytic Study and Treatment of Children," *The Bulletin of the Hampstead Clinic* 1 [1978]:7).

By agreement with the British Psycho-Analytical Society, the Hampstead Clinic was from its inception called the Hampstead Child-Therapy Clinic, although the method of therapy practiced and taught at the clinic was and is that of child psychoanalysis. Students at the clinic fulfill all the requirements of the usual psychoanalytic training program, including a personal analysis of at least four years duration, five times weekly, and undertake the analysis under supervision of a minimum of three psychoanalytic cases. However, in two respects at least the training differs from conventional psychoanalytic training: the patients are children, and except for the first year, the course is full-time. In this book the terms *child analyst* and *child therapist* are used interchangeably.

The Hampstead Clinic differs from the traditional child guidance clinic in that its orientation is wholly psychoanalytic. The bulk of the treatment provided takes the form of full psychoanalysis, in which each child is seen individually, five times a week, for sessions of fifty minutes, over an extended period of time. Work with parents is also undertaken in a variety of contexts. Detailed records are kept at diagnostic and therapeutic levels, and these records form the basis for psychoanalytic research in which both staff members and students participate. A variety of educational and preventive services add further dimensions to both training and research.

Children are treated at the clinic from the age of two. Their problems and disorders cover a broad spectrum, from "neurotic" developmental disturbances to borderline and psychotic behavior. In addition, because of the special research interests of the clinic, a number of children with major disabilities, such as blindness, are offered psychoanalytic therapy.

Over the years at the clinic, despite significant variations and areas of disagreement, a common therapeutic approach has taken shape, a technical and clinical point of view which has been profoundly influenced by the work of Anna Freud. This agreement is probably due to the clinic's basic understanding of childhood disturbances as the child's deviation from a path of normal development. The individual patient is therefore viewed in the context of expectable and age-appropriate psychological, psychosexual, and psychosocial behavior.

The clinic has also developed a particular approach to the collection of child psychoanalytic data for research purposes. The psychoanalytic material contained in the weekly written reports of therapists at the clinic is subjected at regular intervals to a detailed categorization and classification, called "indexing." The procedures for indexing an analytic case, together with categories and definitions, are described in a set of manuals (Joseph Sandler, "The Hampstead Index as an Instrument of Psychoanalytic Research," *International Journal of Psycho-Analysis* 43 [1962]:287–291).

The therapist treating a case carries out the first indexing at least one year after the child has started treatment. Using the manuals as guides, the indexer records, on large filing cards, clinical observations and vignettes that illustrate the relevant categories. The accumulation of indexed material provides the research worker at the clinic with a "collective psychoanalytic memory," which can be viewed, in Anna Freud's words, as "a storehouse of analytic material which places at the disposal of the single thinker and author an abundance of facts gathered by many, thereby transcending the narrow confines of individual experience and extending the possibilities for insightful study, for constructive comparisons between cases, for deductions and generalizations, and finally for extrapolations of theory from clinical therapeutic work" (Preface to John Bolland and Joseph Sandler, *The Hampstead Psychoanalytic Index* [New York: International Universities Press, 1965]).

After years of indexing, it became clear that the material indexed according to the manual titled "Treatment Situation and Technique" covered many of the technical problems encountered in child analysis and could profitably be used for a comprehensive discussion of child psychoanalytic technique. A group was organized at the clinic, under the direction and chairmanship of Joseph Sandler, which met weekly to discuss the manual and the indexed case material. The group included senior staff members, both psychoanalysts and child psychotherapists, as well as students and occasional visitors. Anna Freud took an active part in all of the meetings. No limit was imposed on the number of meetings, which came to an end after two years. Each meeting was tape-recorded and transcribed.

Strict procedures were adopted for the project. Before each meeting all participants were provided with a section of the manual and corresponding examples from the index cards, which served as the basis for discussion. Because the definitions in the manuals were "working definitions" only, there was much to discuss. Often the clinical examples proved inappropriate, which raised issues of practical and theoretical importance. As a matter of policy, the discussions focused on the clinical experience of the participants, with little or no reference made to the voluminous psychoanalytic literature.

This book incorporates the substance of the discussions. Because of their unique interest and importance, Anna Freud's comments appear verbatim. Contributions from the other participants are blended into the text. The indexing instructions from the manual are also included, both to preserve the framework of the original discussion and to explain the nature of the case extracts.

This book does not pretend to be a comprehensive and exhaustive exposition of child psychoanalytic technique, but it is the most extensive commentary on the subject yet produced. It has emerged in its particular form partly because of the format of the discussions and partly because of their reliance on clinical data. The recorded material could not be simply summarized or edited; rather, the points made had to be revamped and reorganized many times. At the same time the text was allowed to retain something of the flavor of the original discussion. Because the recorded material underwent so much synthesis and integration for publication, it has been influenced by the personal views and biases of the authors, who take full responsibility for the text while gratefully acknowledging the contributions of their colleagues.

Part One

The Framework of Treatment

1

Scheduling and Attendance

The importance in psychoanalytic treatment of scheduling five sessions weekly for the patient is a subject of controversy, for psychoanalysis cannot be defined simply on the basis of the number of treatment sessions per week. Yet the number of sessions provided weekly is relevant to the difficult question of the distinction between psychoanalysis and psychotherapy.

ANNA FREUD   Five times a week is the desirable number of attendances for child analysis, and even five hours weekly represents a relatively slight contact with a child. The most intensive contact feasible is needed, not only to gather the maximum amount of material but also to keep the interpretative work going, to keep the analytic material as far as possible within the bounds of the treatment situation, to deal with the anxieties aroused by it and not to place too great a burden on the child's environment. Any lessening of the frequency of attendance for these reasons is detrimental to the efficiency of the analyst's work. Viewed this way, five weekly hours in child analysis is a mere minimum and certainly not a maximum. When psychoanalysis began, the rule, even though for adults, was to have six sessions weekly. It was for social reasons (that is, the introduction of the "weekend") that "daily treatment" has now decreased from six to five sessions a week. In some countries it has dropped to four, or even to three, for a variety of reasons.

To Index: State the agreed number of treatment sessions per week. Describe regularity or irregularity of attendance as well as unpunctuality, and the reasons (e.g. illness, resistance, family problems). Note the degree to which irregular attendance at sessions interferes with treatment.

Five sessions weekly is not a magical number but is the best approximation which can be made to an ideal of daily treatment. In this regard, there is little doubt that economic and financial considerations, on the part of both the patient and the therapist, are important factors in the trend toward the reduction of the number of weekly sessions and of their duration as well. Many therapists have been tempted to maintain that fewer sessions per week are adequate for psychoanalytic work proper. But this is often a rationalization of the wish to take on patients for treatment who cannot afford to pay the therapist's minimum fee five times a week.

ANNA FREUD   If, in the past, a patient could afford only a small fee, this did not alter the belief that he needed his full treatment time. The smaller fee was divided between the requisite number of hours, which meant that the analyst earned less but the patient still received his time. It is a deplorable step in recent developments that now the number of sessions given is usually regulated according to finance instead of according to the conditions favorable for psychoanalysis. But here analysts also meet with a change in people's conventions and attitudes. In the early years of analysis, an analyst who let it be known that he wanted to reduce the treatment frequency for financial reasons would have met with such severe criticism from his colleagues that he would have refrained from doing so.

Sometimes there are reasons other than financial which, at the start of treatment, require the frequency of sessions to be less than five times weekly. For example, a child may live so far away that the analyst chooses to give the child a few sessions weekly rather than none at all. Another reason might be that the child's disturbance is of the sort that five times weekly analysis is not indicated. Such children may not be suitable "control" cases for the purpose of training psychoanalysts.

There is a trend away from the original ideal of "daily" treatment. This trend has been brought about by several factors, including financial pressures, social changes and difficulties that affect children particularly, such as living far away or the special requirements of school and family. It is important to create a model situation of five times a week attendance, with daily sessions of fifty minutes. For purposes of training, there should be no deviation from this arrangement, even though it may sound arbitrary in some respects. It is the best approximation the analyst can make to daily contact, but is in itself not a "definition" of psychoanalysis as opposed to other methods. Psychoanalysis cannot be defined on the basis of frequency of sessions alone.

Whereas these points may hold equally well for adult and for child analysis, there are important differences in child analysis insofar as the child therapist always has to deal with two parties, the patient and the parents. This distinction is easily made when considering the question of payment for the analysis. Not paying the bill is usually looked upon as a sign of the patient's resistance in adult analysis. In child analysis, nonpayment by the parents may be understood as their resistance, or as an expression of their ambivalence, and not as expressing the patient's resistance. In contrast to the treatment of an adult, these attitudes are not necessarily reflected in the child's analytic material. Negative attitudes on the part of the parents may also show themselves in other ways.

ANNA FREUD   The parents of a child under treatment demonstrated their ambivalence to the analysis by not transporting their little boy to the clinic for four whole weeks. At the same time they kept up their financial contributions to make quite sure that his place would not be filled by someone else.

The therapist's own attitudes to missed sessions are important. These attitudes might depend on whether the patient is being seen privately or in a clinic setting. In private practice many child and adult analysts may (and usually do) make arrangements to charge for missed sessions regardless of the reason. In a clinic the therapist's income is not subject to the vagaries of the patient's attendance, and therefore problems of paying fees for missed sessions may not seem so important to the therapist undertaking the analysis. The therapist might therefore more easily collude with either the parents' or the patient's resistance when this resistance is manifested by missing sessions. For the child therapist in such a setting, the special problem is to discern whose resistance accounts for the absence, and whom to confront with the problem of missed sessions.

It may sometimes be useful to take up the matter of fees and paying for missed sessions with the child. In a case treated without fee at the clinic the therapist found it necessary to raise the matter of re- peated missed sessions directly with the child and with the father. Both father and patient were told that the treatment did in fact cost money, and that someone had to pay for the missed sessions even if they did not. Afterward the attendance improved, though the un- conscious reasons for the patient's difficulties in attending were not analyzed at that point.

ANNA FREUD   If children learn about the money paid for treatment, they always feel that this is a terrific waste, and they do so whether their feelings toward the analyst and analysis are positive or nega- tive. A young boy patient of mine used to calculate how many tracks for his electric railway he would be able to buy for a single hour's fee. If given the choice, there is no doubt that he would have preferred the tracks to the analytic hour, in spite of his good treatment alliance and positive transference.

The child's feelings about the value of treatment may be known to the parents, as in one situation where the family tended to think of values chiefly in terms of money. They were aware that their latency son echoed these sentiments, and they insisted they be allowed to tell their son how much the analytic fee was, so that he would have greater respect for the treatment. The child's age plays an important part in the degree to which treatment may be valued in terms of money, as a very young child has no conception of the meaning of money.

Often parents value the treatment less than the therapist thinks they should. Some seem to feel that child analysis is, in the last re- sort, no more than "play" and, for this reason, should be less expen- sive than analysis for adults. Another possible factor is that parents are accustomed to paying half-fare for their children on railroads and buses. All sorts of social and personal factors influence the value that parents place on the child's treatment, and these are not neces- sarily directly related to what they pay for it.

ANNA FREUD   There are many cases where analysts understand the need for the child's treatment while the parents are ignorant of it or only pay lip service to it. However, it is a mistake to forget that the final decision rests with the parents, just as in adult analysis it rests with the patient himself. A child's analysis, not sufficiently wanted or valued by the parents, will come to grief at some point. We at the clinic perhaps err on the side of urging treatment of the child when the parents themselves do not feel sufficiently positive about it. I personally take the parents' signs of unwillingness or indecision as seriously as I do such signs with adults who have to decide about their own treatment. Some parents seem extremely eager during the initial interviews, and are even offended if no vacancy can be offered immediately, only to change their attitude as soon as treatment has begun. Music lessons, riding lessons, the social contact of the child with friends will then be used as excuses for missed sessions. Obviously, in these instances the analysts have not taken into account the parents' low valuation of analysis, their conscious and unconscious resistances. This can be as destructive for the child's analysis as it is for adult analysis, where the decision to undergo treatment has not been left exclusively to the individual's own wishes.

The parents' apparent unwillingness may represent only an initial and superficial resistance, and it is possible to win the parents over. A great deal depends on whether the child's symptoms are "parent-syntonic" (cause no trouble and are acceptable to the parents) or are a source of real pain and discomfort to the parents. When the therapist looks at the problem from the point of view of the child's development, he may be much more aware of the gravity and urgency of the difficulties.

In one case the child's resistance to treatment was shown by missing sessions. Katrina L., who was six years and one month old when analytic treatment began, was indexed at the age of seven years and one month:

During her first year of treatment Katrina missed some eight weeks altogether, the longest break of three and one-half weeks being when Katrina contracted measles. Other interruptions of variable length occurred because of illnesses, minor ailments, holidays, or refusal to come to her session. It seemed that, illnesses and external events aside, it was in reality Katrina's resistances which determined the length and frequency of her absences. This also showed itself in her chronic lateness for sessions during the first half year of treatment, which came about because of her delaying tactics when it was time to leave home. During the second half of that year, Katrina's lateness decreased considerably and she attended regularly, although she often threatened not to come.

ANNA FREUD   Child patients have many ways of expressing their negative reactions to interpretation and to other analytic interventions. These reactions range from verbal expression of anger to leaving the treatment room for shorter or longer periods, running to the toilet, to the waiting room, and so on. There is a whole continuum of responses, from the mere threat "never to come again," which is not carried out, to the actual refusal to come. It is not the children who threaten to stay away who actually discontinue attendance. What is expressed verbally does not need to be converted into action.

It is not always possible to differentiate sharply between internal resistances and reality factors, though as therapists, we attempt this. The connections between attendance and resistance, both in the child and in the parent, show up in the case of Susan S. Susan began treatment at the age of three, and her case was indexed when she was six years and six months old. She entered treatment because of emotional disturbances associated with constitutional sexual precocity (Ruth Thomas, with Lydia Folkart and Elizabeth Model, "The Search for a Sexual Identity in a Case of Constitutional Sexual Precocity," *The Psychoanalytic Study of the Child* 18 [1963]).

For the first year, Susan was seen three times a week because her mother would not bring her more often. Eventually the mother agreed to bring her five times a week. In the third year of treatment, for a period of three months Susan would only stay in the waiting room, but the analytic work continued as the therapist joined her there. This was a sort of compromise between attending and not attending.

Susan had in fact a treatment alliance which allowed the analytic work to continue in spite of the apparent resistance and conflict over attending which kept her in the waiting room so long. In another and older child not brought by the parent, the resistance might have resulted in missed sessions. The case illustrates the effect of the mother's and the child's conflict over coming to treatment, as shown by the mother's initial refusal to bring her daughter more than thrice weekly, and then by Susan's period of staying in the waiting room.

Helen D. provides an example of striking regularity in attendance.

She was twelve years old when treatment began, and fifteen when the case was indexed:

Helen's unfailing attendance continued throughout treatment. There were periods when she felt hostile to the analyst and she threatened to leave the clinic immediately and never to come again. In fact she never did walk out nor did she ever miss a session, because her defensive need to cling to the object was heightened by becoming aware of her anger.

ANNA FREUD The behavior of this girl suggests the diagnosis. She behaves in an obsessional way because of her ambivalence and the whole obsessional arrangement of her personality. Such children remain highly conscientious about attending, even during periods of negative transference. They continue to come in the same way, even if they threaten to break off and express their wishes to leave. This example illustrates a reason for the regularity of attendance, which is an outcome of the child's pathology. It reminds me of a girl in analysis with a colleague of mine. The patient made no treatment alliance and she was in a negative transference toward her analyst. This child did not want to cooperate, but one day the arrangement for bringing her from school broke down and she ran all the way from school to her analyst's house, arrived breathless and on time, and started her usual resistance. Her regularity reflected only her obsessional conscientiousness, and it was neither transference nor treatment alliance.

This kind of obsessionality can also be seen in young children as a reflection of a parent's obsessionality about regularity. The child arrives at every session on time and without absences simply because he is brought by the parent. Other parental attitudes might be reflected in a child's variations in attendance.

ANNA FREUD Unpunctuality and irregularity in attendance may be due to either the child's or the parents' attitude. On the part of the child it can reflect either something inherent in his character and pathology, or something inherent in the transference and treatment alliance. In the parents it can reflect either something in their whole attitude to life and their way of life (for example, a Bohemian tendency, chronic unpunctuality, chronic inability to stick to a contract), or a special hostility to analysis or to the child's welfare.

Certainly therapists vary in their attitudes toward attendance and missed sessions. A particular attitude of the therapist is probably communicated early in treatment in one way or another, and it may allow for the parental exploitation of the therapist's leniency or laxness in regard to attendance. For instance, some therapists very readily agree to changing appointment times while others do not. Similarly, there are parents who make frequent use of external events to cancel sessions and others with whom it happens only rarely.

In child analysis the therapist must always take into account the importance of reality events in the patient's life. For example, examinations or school outings do interfere with attendance. With adults the analyst can take up an easier stance, saying simply that the sessions are there and have to be paid for; it is up to the patient what use he makes of them. The therapist cannot take a rigid and inflexible position about the child's attending but has to consider the external circumstances of both the patient and the parents. One must balance the reality situation against the need for continuity of treatment.

ANNA FREUD   I remember from my own practice the situation of an older schoolgirl who was under great pressure during examination time. My inclination was to give her time off from analysis, whereas the parents were insistent that no treatment should be missed. Accordingly, the girl appeared dutifully for her sessions but little useful analytic work was done. Differences of opinion of this kind are not easy to resolve, and judgments vary also among analysts as to what is reasonable.

The therapist must allow a certain amount of leeway from the ideal situation as defined in the basic rule. For example, the therapist may allow a child to come ten minutes late once a week when some special school activity makes it awkward to be on time. Or the therapist may agree that the child leave his daily early morning session five minutes early in order to arrive at school on time so as to avoid the embarrassment of coming late or the scathing remarks of a hostile teacher. However, if after a long period of time the analysis is not going well, one may well ask whether or not this arrangement has become a resistance. That which at the outset was a reality problem might have come to be utilized by the forces of resistance.

Many adolescents in treatment tend to get involved in outside activities, in their schooling, hobbies, and other aspects of their external lives, which interfere with the time of their analytic sessions. Adolescents may still not come to treatment the prescribed number of times despite analysis of their resistances. However, the therapist should be aware that in all the adolescent's activities which interfere with the analysis there may be an expression of the adolescent's struggle to break the infantile ties to the parents. It is important not to fall into the pattern of automatically interpreting all such activities as resistance and thus reinforcing the infantile ties and dependencies against which the adolescent fights. Another consequence of an "automatic" interpretation of resistance in this situation is to stimulate the adolescent's resistance so that treatment has to be broken off.

ANNA FREUD   In the case of children and adolescents the claims of analysis and of normal progressive development do not always coincide. What is good for the one may be detrimental for the other. An example is the child patient on the border between early infantile and latency development. For the purpose of analysis, conscious access to the pregenital strivings has to be kept open; for the purpose of latency development, the infantile amnesia should set in and the past be closed off by repression and the use of other defenses. Similarly, in adolescence the need for growing independence clashes with the analytic need for reawakening past dependency in the transference.

The view that missing sessions might, in certain cases, act as a "safety valve" is a controversial one. Therapists should not advocate the missing of sessions, despite the fact that occasional absences can have a "protective" function.

Certain adolescents, especially those who are afraid of the intense feelings involved in an attachment to the therapist, would show less resistance in analysis if they were to attend for less than the usual five times a week.

ANNA FREUD   As regards adolescents, I agree that their fear of analysis is lessened if the demands on attendance are lessened, but it is not usual analytic policy to lessen anxieties by avoiding their arousal. Perhaps the best analogy in this respect is the fear of the couch with certain adult patients whose passive and homosexual trends are aroused when they have to assume the lying-down position. It is true that they are reassured if permitted to sit in a chair, but it is also true that under these conditions neither the passivity nor the homosexuality will come into the analysis. It is as if analysts allowed the patient to say, "I am willing to be analyzed so long as certain areas of my pathology are not touched on."

Regularity of attendance may have a meaning which is often missed precisely because the patient attends regularly. There are patients who place importance on arriving regularly and on time, but who do not place the same value on doing analytic work. In some cases, frequent and regular attendance is accompanied by endless repetition, and all the relevant material in the week could perhaps have been brought up in one session. However, the idea that fewer sessions weekly would be more efficient, because there would be fewer sessions of resistance, is wishful thinking. What is important is to be in sufficiently frequent contact with the child in order to be able to conduct the analytic work.

2

Interruptions

The patient's reactions to interruptions can be extremely meaningful to the therapist for they highlight the stages of development reached by the child and the points to which he regresses, as well as his pathology. The child has a variety of responses to normal and unexpected interruptions, with which the therapist has to deal.

Vacations and holidays can be regarded as normal interruptions. Even if the therapist's or the clinic's vacation time does not coincide with school vacation, many children tend to equate periods of going to school ("term time") with coming to treatment. The reason for this equation lies in the fact that both school and treatment are arrangements made for them by the parents, and they are expected to attend whether they find the experience pleasant or unpleasant, interesting or frightening. When the therapist's and the school's vacations do not coincide, the child's feelings often appear in the analytic material and may be taken up in treatment.

ANNA FREUD There has always been lively discussion of the question of whether a holiday from school, such as half-term, should automatically imply a holiday from therapy. When I have advocated this practice in order to avoid unnecessary battles with the child patient, many therapists have taken an opposite point of view. Obviously some therapists do not take kindly to the idea that children consider analysis to be a duty imposed on them by

To Index: Describe the child's reactions to interruptions of treatment, for whatever cause (e.g. planned or regular interruptions such as holidays and weekends, therapist's absence for any reason). Describe anticipatory reactions as well as those occurring after the interruption.

the outside world just as the duty to go to school is imposed. However, while there are many children who insist on their right to spend a day free from school on activities of their own choosing, and who do not appear for their session at the school half-term holiday even if the analyst wishes them to do so, there are others whose attitude is different. They are often children who are tied to the analyst as a real person, as if he were a substitute parent from whom they do not want to be separated. Every interruption of analysis is treated by them as if it meant an interruption of the parent-child relationship; that is, it makes them feel neglected and rejected.

Some therapists whose vacations do not coincide with school vacations want their patients to come to treatment when on vacation from school, but having a battle over this may turn the child against the idea of treatment, arousing unnecessary resistance and resentment against what the child feels to be an intrusion on a well-deserved break. One way of dealing with this problem is to say to the patient, "I am not on vacation at this time and am available for you if you want to come," which might allow the patient's conflict over therapy to be brought into the analysis. There is also much to be said for the view that the therapist should not expect the child, especially the younger child, to want to come during the school vacations. Although, quite understandably, most child patients resent having to attend their analytic sessions when other children have the whole day free, there are exceptions, particularly children who have a strong motivation for treatment and are very aware of the painful nature of their symptoms. The wish of the child to have a "day off" from analysis is similar to the reaction sometimes seen in children of nonreligious parents who have to go to school when most of their friends are out because of a religious holiday: they feel that they are being forced to do something they have a right not to do. The wish to stay away from treatment during a school holiday *may* be an expression of resistance, but it is quite clear that not all wishes to stay away during holidays originate thus.

ANNA FREUD   I have always wanted to make an experiment in the clinic, though one cannot do such things. It would be, let us say, that during a certain week only those children should come for treatment who really wanted to come on their own, without any pressure from anybody else. I don't say there would be none, but you'd be surprised how few there *would* be.

Even though it is not always easy to distinguish reality reasons from other reasons, it is worth making the effort in order to verify interpretations of resistance. Certainly the emergence of resistance to the analytic work may sometimes utilize a coming holiday, and the patient's wish not to come can be interpreted as resistance in this context.

A danger exists in the too consistent interpretation of reactions to interruptions as expressions of resistance. After all, if the child is angry on a Monday, it cannot automatically be inferred that the child is angry because he was not seen on the weekend. It might be more fitting at times to interpret the child's anger as related to his having had to return to treatment. It is extremely difficult to distinguish between reality-based reasons and resistance in both child and adult patients. Some therapists deal with the difficulty by treating any wish not to come as resistance or by taking refuge in a "strict" analytic posture.

Those children who agree, or want, to come to treatment during school holidays often request a change of time, which, for reality reasons, may be entirely appropriate for either patient or therapist or both. Making the appointment at a more convenient time may offer a solution to the child's conflict over coming to his sessions during a holiday. The change of time may disengage the treatment from its equation with school.

The reaction of the child to an interruption in treatment must always be examined in the context of the state of his analysis at that time. The importance of the analytical context is illustrated by the case of a child who had previously accepted and adapted to weekend breaks and holidays during his analysis. Suddenly, in the third year of his treatment, he reacted to the routine interruption in a way reminiscent of his reaction to the first holiday break in his analysis. The analytic material made it clear that this reaction represented a repetition of a separation which had occurred much earlier in his life. His reaction in the third year of his analysis could only be understood in terms of what was going on in his analysis: the current revival of fears of separation and loss in the transference. Other types of reaction may be determined by the predominant mode of defense, as in the case of the child who regularly misses a session either after or before a holiday, making use of the mechanism of turning passive into active. By missing the session, he does to the therapist what he feels was done to him.

Another determinant of reactions to interruptions is the level of the child's object relation to the therapist. An example is the child (or adult) who is unable to come to a session for some reason and then reacts as if the therapist were the one who had canceled the session. It is the separation from the therapist rather than the cause of the separation which is important for the patient.

The problem also arises of how to deal with sessions canceled by the therapist.

ANNA FREUD   When I have to cancel sessions or when I have to travel, I find it simplest to give the patients the reason for my absence. However, this does not prevent them from substituting their fantasies for the reality reason which they have been offered. For example, I may explain that I am going somewhere for purposes of work; when I return, the patient may nevertheless say that he hopes I have had an enjoyable holiday. It means that, so far as he is concerned, I have taken a holiday from working with him.

Although the patient may be told why the therapist has to cancel a session, the explanation should be put in general terms, without too many details. Nevertheless, patients of any age often react badly to an unexpected and unexplained cancellation. Often the therapist may bring something of his problems to such situations. He may deal with his guilt feelings, for example, by saying each time that he is sorry, by declaring his helplessness, or by feeling obliged to offer long explanations or to make up sessions missed. Alternatively, the therapist may go to the opposite extreme by rigidly adhering to analytic "rules" and thus fail to handle the realistic aspects of the situation.

ANNA FREUD   Sometimes the interruption is especially difficult for the patient, and it is best to acknowledge that. I said to a patient, and I really meant it, "You know, I am sorry we have to interrupt just now. I would not have chosen this moment. I think it is a very unfortunate one." The patient knows that there are commitments, or trips, or even holidays which cannot be changed at a moment's notice. But it helps the situation if one acknowledges it. The worst thing is to remain neutral and offer no explanation.

A break may sometimes be acceptable, or may even be a relief to the patient, if it interrupts a sterile period in the analytic work. The therapist may even wish to introduce small breaks into the analytic routine quite deliberately in order to stimulate the patient to do more productive analytic work on returning to treatment.

ANNA FREUD   Many years ago this problem was discussed under the heading of "fractionated analysis," a term which implied that patients would benefit from doing some "working-through" on their own. It did not usually work out in practice with either adults or with children. The resistances were often greatly strengthened in the interval and resulted in an absolute unwillingness to return to therapy in spite of the patient still being in need of treatment.

Certain children seem to make progressive developmental steps during vacation breaks. Particularly with latency children changes may be noted after a vacation which may be interpreted as a distancing from instinctual conflict and the beginning of sublimation, but which may actually be part of a sealing-up process that is expected in latency.

ANNA FREUD   It is very much a question of the type of illness treated. With the very severely ill child, either borderline or autistic, holidays are usually disastrous. There is a complete loss of therapeutic gain, which is quite different from what happens with neurotic children during holidays. Whoever works with borderline children has had the experience of losing the child as a patient during a holiday interruption. The same is true of adult addicts and alcoholics who, in my experience, benefit from analysis only if analytic contact is kept up without any Sunday or holiday break. In the neurotic patient, the effects of interruption were discussed many years ago in the context of the "Monday crust," the hardening of resistances which analysts met in their patients after the Sunday interruption. We can expect an even harder "crust" now, when we have a two-day interruption at weekends. We cannot be certain what sort of "crust" will form in an analysis involving only three or four sessions a week. This problem is relevant to the issue of the differences between psychoanalysis and psychotherapy and the relation of these differences to frequency of sessions.

Many technical problems are posed for the therapist by interruptions. An interruption may revive a traumatic experience, necessitating special handling if it is believed that the traumatic experience (particularly of separation) is significant for the child's pathology. Another issue is the technical problem of whether to maintain the analytic relationship with the child, by telephone or by written contact, during absences or breaks. Children's individual sensitivity to interruptions may present problems. Certain children react strongly to the interruption between one session and another, or to the weekend breaks. A summer vacation, for a very young child, may be equivalent to a break of a much longer duration for an adult, because the very young child may not have developed sufficient object-constancy for the therapist to retain a meaningful role in the child's inner world over a prolonged vacation.

A typical case is that of Jerry N., who began treatment at the age of four years four months; his material was indexed when he was six years four months:

In the course of treatment it became apparent that Jerry reacted with anxiety and rage to any kind of break in treatment or separation from the therapist. Jerry was a child who had never actually been separated from his mother, but his mother was depressed during his early years and also during his analysis. Her depression was manifested by withdrawal from and hostility toward her husband and her children. Jerry always demanded a detailed explanation of unplanned interruptions. Even with planned holidays Jerry's reactions included fantasies both before and after the holiday that the therapist might die or be damaged when away from him. After the therapist had been away because of illness, Jerry brought the fantasy that he would break the clinic down, destroying the therapist's room. After holidays he was messy and angry and took some time to settle down.

A link is apparent between the mother's depression, experienced by Jerry as a hostile act, and Jerry's anxious fantasies about separation in treatment, although the situation with the mother was revived and repeated in the transference in acute form only at times of separation because of holidays or illness.

Another case involved a latency boy, Quentin J., who began treatment aged nine years one month; his case was indexed when he was ten years four months:

> In his first year of treatment, the most important aspect of interruptions of treatment for Quentin was related to feelings of deprivation. In his second year, after considerable analytic work, his orientation toward separations in the analysis shifted. He had grown two hyacinth bulbs, and he brought these to the last session before a holiday, saying they were a present for the therapist. He asked especially that she should take them home with her for the holiday but bring them back to the treatment room afterward.

This case illustrates a step in the line of development of object relations; after "I want to keep you with me," the next step is "I want you to keep me with you." Sometimes a child insists on taking something home from treatment, but in this example the patient wanted the therapist to keep something.

A child can respond to a separation in many different ways, which may illustrate different stages in the development of the child's object relationships. For example, one girl of thirteen, during a certain phase of the analysis, found it difficult to cope with the daily separations from the therapist and expressed the wish that the therapist should follow her to school as if she were her shadow. She later brought the wishful fantasy that the therapist should sculpt her patients; she herself subsequently made a plasticine figure of mother and baby in her session. The therapist was asked to look after it until the next day.

Nine-year-old Freddy, in a similar phase in his analysis, brought a caterpillar in a matchbox to a session and expressed the wish to put the therapist into that box and carry her with him in his pocket wherever he went. Another child wanted to bring animals for the therapist to look after. He frantically insisted, "You must take that dog! No one wants it, no one looks after it. I will bring it tomorrow and you must look after it."

A nine-year-old girl looked into her therapist's eyes and said, "I can see myself in your eyes." She put her hands over the therapist's face and said, "I could make a model of you and then I'd have it there." She put a bit of wool into a locket which the therapist had to wear around her neck and subsequently checked whether this bit of wool was inside whenever the therapist wore the locket.

A four-year-old boy was very angry at the impending separation for the holidays. To help him with his feelings about losing her, the therapist wrote down her name and holiday address; during the session the boy ate the piece of paper on which this information was written, thus symbolically keeping the therapist with him.

Certainly a child's past experiences related to separation and to other aspects of the early relationship to the parents enter into the child's responses to separations in treatment. The child's fantasies about the causes and meanings of the interruption, and his anticipatory and actual responses, are affected not only by his level of object relationship but also by the nature of his pathology and the current state of the transference. This point is useful in understanding the reactions of the borderline child, who may fear that if he cannot actually perceive the object, it no longer exists.

ANNA FREUD   There are other reactions which occur at a slightly higher developmental level. For example, a three-and-one-half-year-old boy in the Hampstead Nurseries, after separation from his mother the first evening, said that he had to telephone her that night because she would be so sad. This means that he did not emphasize his own feelings of sadness and separation. This is not necessarily a defense against his feelings of sadness. People tend always to consider the wish to keep a love object near to them as a one-sided process. However, the other wish, to be kept in mind by the loved object, can be equally strong. Few child patients would mind an interruption in the analysis if they could feel sure that the analyst was sitting in his room thinking of them.

Although children often attempt to use a symbolic way of maintaining contact with the therapist during a break, the critical factor is not so much whether the patient loves or hates the therapist during the break in treatment as whether the therapist and treatment are sufficiently invested with importance until sessions begin again.

Children sometimes show a greater tendency than adults to "seal up" during an interruption.

ANNA FREUD   I remember a girl of six who came back after a long summer break of nearly three months. She started exactly as if she had been there the day before, and interruption had changed nothing. She had probably, according to her individual nature, continued the relationship right through the break. Whether she did so in actual fantasy conversations I do not know, but when I showed my surprise that we had played a game not yesterday but three months ago, she answered, "But do you think that my coming here is something that I can forget just like that?" However, in other cases, or if the break has come in the phase where something negative was uppermost, one would get exactly the opposite impression: children may act as if they had never seen the analyst before.

The common statement of therapists that a child had a "marked reaction" to separation or interruption in treatment tells remarkably little. The question arises as to what the reaction was. Did the child show resistance? Did he show anger? Did he simply express one or another fantasy? One should distinguish between the child's anticipatory reactions, his reactions during the course of the separation (in order to maintain contact, to deny feelings, and so on), and the expression of his feelings about the interruption when treatment resumes. The child's reactions to interruptions are like responses to a psychological test which measures the changes in a child during the course of the analysis. On the one hand, the child adapts to the analytic process over a number of years, and on the other, actual changes in the child occur as a consequence of the analytic work and the developmental process.

3

Change of Therapist

In child psychoanalysis a change of therapist is to be avoided. Ideally the therapist should be changed only if there are good clinical grounds. Unfortunately at a training institute it is frequently necessary to change a patient's therapist since the student therapists leave at the end of training, which gives the problem special importance.

Among the reasons it is disadvantageous to change analysts is the disruption which occurs both in the child's relationship to the therapist and in the treatment alliance. Although it might be thought that the child would find it easier than an adult to accept a substitute therapist because of the child's greater readiness to enter into a variety of new relationships, in fact children normally get as upset as adults at having to make a change. Indeed, a change of therapist might be more difficult for a child patient than for an adult because the child's attachment to the therapist as a real person is usually greater than that of the adult patient. Of course there is a variation from one patient to another, and it is difficult to compare children in general with adults in this context.

It is understandable that a child may object to a change of therapist imposed "from above," especially if the relationship to the previous therapist has been a good one and useful analytic work has been done. The greatest objections may come from those children for whom a gratifying real relationship with the therapist has been the most important ingredient in their sessions together. A relatively

To Index: Indicate the date a change of therapist occurred, the point in treatment, the reason, and the child's reactions. Describe the way in which the changeover was organized and the child prepared. Include the child's responses to both the anticipated and the actual change.

26

mature reaction can be seen in children who, after initial objection and working-through, are able to distinguish between the function of the therapist as a real person and his function as a therapist.

ANNA FREUD   It is the relationship on the basis of object constancy which comes into question when the change of therapist is objected to. I had occasion to hear about the opposite reaction for the first time in the Tegelsee Sanatorium in Berlin where alcoholics and other addicts were under treatment; these were patients who could be analyzed only while living in a protected, residential environment. It was reported in a case seminar to everybody's surprise that substitution of the analyst did not seem to matter. When a patient's analyst had his day off, another analyst could go into the patient's room, sit down, and conduct an analytic session with him. Obviously, the addict's transference relationship was based on a level below object constancy—namely on need fulfillment, so that it was not the person of the object which mattered, merely his function. This was convenient for the management of the sanatorium but throws a sinister light on the level of object relations to be found in certain addicts.

In some institutional settings there is a conscious effort to encourage the development of a relationship at the need-satisfying (part object) level, that is, to a constantly changing set of staff members (usually nurses) whose role is indicated by a uniform. Many patients develop transferences to the institution as well as to a specific person. Many clinic patients show a relationship to the clinic as a whole, or sometimes a special relationship to such people as the waiting room receptionist, besides the special relationship to the therapist. In certain patients an exaggeration of the relationship to auxiliary personnel may represent a defensive withdrawal from closeness to the therapist. The patient defends by diffusing the relationship throughout the institution. This is quite different from a displacement of transference feelings to a specific "other" person within the institution.

The level of object relationships to which a child has developed must be considered when attempting to understand the nature of the child's reactions to a change of therapist. The therapist must ask whether the reactions represent feelings of broken trust, responses of anger and resentment at a reality loss, or links with and revivals of past experiences of object loss.

ANNA FREUD   An interesting example of this problem is a severely ill twenty-year-old boy who had been in psychoanalytic psychotherapy and had finally made a good attachment to and treatment alliance with one of the psychiatrists. He had improved somewhat, but he was still in the middle of his treatment when the psychiatrist changed jobs and left town. The boy made plans to follow him, because for the first time in his life he felt that treatment helped him and he wanted to continue. In the case discussion, his behavior was thought to be abnormal and irrational in his wanting to follow his doctor. I would have taken it as a sign that the treatment relationship had acquired meaning in his life, that he was not ready to let go of it, and that he would not accept in what might be called a promiscuous way the same relationship with a successor.

A complicated and intricate link exists between separation anxiety and reactions to change of therapist. For those children who seem to accept the prospective change of therapist quite easily, acceptance may be a sign of mental health rather than of pathological object relationships. If a proper relationship to the therapist had developed, however, the child would want to continue with that therapist and would show distress at the idea of going to someone else. A successful changeover requires that the child establish a treatment relationship with the new therapist and recognize as well that he is relating to a different person from the previous therapist.

The case of Michael B. illustrates a child's reaction to change of therapist. Michael's treatment began when he was five years and ten months old, and his material was indexed at seven years and eight months:

Michael was in analysis with his first therapist for a year, following which his therapist returned to his own country in July. In September, after the vacation, Michael commenced analysis with his second therapist, with whom he remained until treatment was terminated two years later. Michael had intense reactions to the change of therapist. He had transferred to his second therapist the expectation of being abandoned, as he had been many times early in life by his mother, by *au pair* girls to whom he was attached, and most recently by his first therapist. As a consequence, Michael's developing positive transference feelings toward the second therapist had to be continually defended against and warded off, but together with the therapist he could analyze many of the separations he had experienced, discussing the most recent ones and working back to his earlier losses.

Michael's need to protect himself against developing a relationship with his second therapist was certainly a reflection of his earlier separation experiences, which had been reinforced by loss of the first therapist. He seemed to have gained the conviction that new relationships were not worthwhile because they inevitably led to the pain of loss. Although this problem posed difficulties in the treatment situation, of necessity it became the focus of the analytic work leading to the analysis and working-through of Michael's problems of repeated separation and loss.

Change of therapist creates a real situation onto which the transference reactions can be latched. As a real situation, it may revive significant childhood experiences amenable to analysis. These situations are not intentionally set up, but when they occur, their effects can be taken up in the analysis both from the side of reality and from the side of the reactions and fantasies brought by the patient.

When the analysis has not been going well, the loss of the therapist may be a great relief to the child. This is particularly the case when a negative transference has been concealed and not analyzed. The child may then feel obliged to appear "distressed" because of guilt feelings, but may in reality be extremely relieved and looking forward to the changeover. This probably occurs much more often than is realized. In such a case, the child may work very well with a new therapist.

Occasionally change of therapist is a deliberate strategy in treatment, as exemplified by the case of a very big and violent fifteen-year-old boy whose treatment was not going well.

ANNA FREUD   This was a highly disturbed delinquent boy who was given a young therapist of small build and who was seen at a time when the clinic was almost deserted. I am quite sure that he developed the fantasy that he could easily kill the analyst or damage her, and he could have done so. She had the same feeling, and we ended this situation and handed him over to an older and more experienced therapist where the whole thing did not recur. He did marvelously well, but he went through a period of great guilt because of the previous therapist's disappearance. He thought he had actually killed her; it was quite an interesting transfer. It was a mistake in the original allocation, but certainly such mismatches occur.

Although some therapists might take the view that the patient's fantasy of being able to damage the therapist, as well as his overt response to the therapist, could be dealt with by analysis and appropriate interpretation, this is not always possible. In cases where interpretation might be effective with an adult patient, a similar interpretation in a similar situation with an adolescent or child patient might not be effective.

Children have much less to do with choosing or changing their therapists than do adults. Both children and adults often express disappointment at not being in treatment with the therapist who saw them for the diagnostic interview. To get away from a disliked analyst, a child may have to stay away from the session or persuade his parents to break off the analysis. Children express the wish to change therapists for a variety of reasons.

ANNA FREUD   Just as a patient wishes for the constancy of the analyst as an object, there is also a constant wish for a change. With every bit of hostile feeling that comes up there is the wish to go somewhere else. I know it so well from adult analysis. Never, in my experience, have any of my adult patients ever met another analyst without wishing to change over to him or her. When I was a young analyst, I shared a waiting room with my father, which meant that his patients saw me when I fetched mine and my patients saw him. I complained bitterly that it was made so difficult for me, that all my patients wanted to go to him. And he said, "Never mind, all my patients want to go to you." Which is the reason, of course, we are wary about considering the patient's wish for change as an incentive for action; if we did, we would have to change continually.

An enormous difficulty faces the therapist when the child repeatedly expresses, over a long period, a wish to have a different therapist. This wish can be looked at simply as a manifestation of a severe resistance, and the therapist can attempt to analyze it as part of the analytic work. There are other cases, however, in which the reluctance to attend, even though based on the child's neurotic conflicts, is so great that a change of therapist might be indicated in the hope that the next therapist might be able to work it through. Therapists also have to face the fact that some patients continue in resistance simply because their therapists have been unable to reach an effective understanding of the material. Here too the solution might well be a change of therapist.

The child's reaction to a change of therapist might depend on whether the child himself is in transition from one phase of the analysis to another. The example of Kenny K. is apposite here. This patient had a strong attachment to his first analyst, with whom he began treatment at the age of six years and three months; the transfer to his second therapist occurred just at the point where the patient was ready to begin the working-through process and the abandonment of his symptoms. The second therapist indexed the case when Kenny was nine years and three months old. The child had originally been referred for treatment because of soiling:

Kenny had two years of treatment with a male therapist and then changed over to a female therapist because the first analyst left the country. Kenny was told of the change two months beforehand. He anxiously inquired about the successor and seemed to feel betrayed that it should be a woman, whom he at first refused to meet. He thought his therapist was leaving him because he had not stopped soiling, and his presenting symptom remained until some time after the changeover. He started treatment with his new therapist after a long summer holiday. At first he was polite, yet he revealed some of his problems quickly. He had to compare his new therapist's competence by playing checkers with her; he denied his sad and angry feelings about his former therapist but enacted them in symbolic play together with his fears of punishment. Gradually he came to establish a relationship with the new therapist and to express fantasies of having been given a better mother. Following this, additional analytic work around the soiling symptom became possible, and the symptom disappeared.

Kenny had refused to meet the new therapist before the vacation, claiming to feel betrayed that he was being transferred to a woman therapist. The change of therapist may in fact have been unconsciously welcomed by Kenny, as indicated by his later fantasy of being given a better mother, but he felt very guilty about this. It is also possible that the wish for a "better mother" might have appeared in treatment with the first therapist if that therapist had remained. In Kenny's case the changeover was from a male student to

a more experienced woman staff member, which may have influenced the later progress of the case.

ANNA FREUD   We at the clinic transfer cases from a less experienced
to a more experienced analyst, because of our awareness of the
difficulties involved in changeovers. We have had cases in which
the second analyst was more successful than the first, but I have
the impression that this can be related either to the change from a
man to a woman therapist, or vice versa, or to changing to a more
experienced therapist. We also have many examples of children
who have never forgiven what they felt to be an abandonment and
breach of trust, and the analytic work has had to end.

For training purposes it is preferable not to assign a case to a student when the case has been in analytic treatment before. The rationale is that it is advantageous to learn psychoanalytic technique
without having to deal with the complicated problems that a changeover entails. The student should, however, receive supervised experience of handling such problems.

The situations that arise in regard to change of therapist fall into
three groups. First, there are those situations where the change is
made very smoothly by the child, on the basis of the child's need for
therapeutic help and the relief which the child receives, providing
that the new therapist functions effectively. Another group of children present considerable difficulties in coping with the change of
therapist, experiencing long periods of sadness and distress which
have to be worked through with the new therapist. And finally, there
are those children for whom the change of therapist is disastrous for
the analysis, so that work with the new therapist never gets off the
ground. It is extremely important to realize that a failure to make a
successful change of therapist may occur even though the new
therapist is highly skilled.

When a therapist has to leave, the situation must be evaluated extremely carefully. It has to be decided whether a termination of analysis is indicated because the child can cope on his own without analysis, or whether transfer to another therapist is preferable. Parental
attitudes and wishes have to be taken into account as well. For some
children a planned termination is obviously most suitable, whereas
for others it is equally obvious that treatment must continue with

another therapist. In the many cases where neither course is clearly indicated it may be advantageous to allow the child to have a break between ending analysis with one therapist and beginning with another, leaving open the options for handling the changeover. Thus the child can have a long summer break before being introduced to any new therapist; after the vacation the child and family may feel that all is well and further therapy is unnecessary. With very disturbed children and with those in whom there is definite evidence that the therapeutic task is far from complete, it is preferable to recommend that the patient have a new therapist to whom he be introduced before the first therapist leaves.

Many child analyses terminate when the therapist has to leave or when the child has to move. The question that should be asked at this point is whether the child can cope without further analytic help. Other terminations occur when the child has progressed to a new developmental phase, one of the signs of this movement being a wish to stop analysis. Again, the question should be asked at this point whether or not the child can manage on his own. The aim of child analysis should be borne in mind in both these cases: to restore the child to the path of normal development.

The preparation of a child for change of therapist or termination of analysis can be handled in several ways. The child can be told about the proposed change as soon as it becomes known to the therapist. There are obvious advantages to this approach for the therapist who might otherwise feel guilty if he kept the termination date secret. Although in some cases setting a date can speed up the analytic work, experience shows that too much advance notice (say, twelve months) may simply arrest the analytic work. It is difficult to make rules about such matters. The therapist must judge, on a clinical basis, whether a long advance warning will be to the benefit of the analysis or not. Once the child has been told of termination, all the various possibilities for the future should be discussed fully with him so that he is not left in a state of unverbalized uncertainty.

The second therapist faces problems. She does not always know the nature of the events in the first or preceding treatment, even if written records are available. Indeed, in private practice it probably happens relatively frequently that the second therapist does not know very much about the previous treatment; this may or may not be an advantage for the work. If the child is seen at a clinic, the institution may provide some continuity for the child who changes therapist, a continuity that is not normally available in private practice. Since the external milieu remains relatively stable, the child may derive some support during the changeover. The therapist must also deal with her own feelings about the changeover. Whereas a therapist who is leaving may feel guilty, sad, inadequate, or envious of a successor, the new therapist may experience competitiveness or fears of disappointing the child. She has also to deal with her feelings about taking on a "secondhand" case.

It is not always easy for the child to work through feelings connected with the change of therapist while the change is still in prospect. Such working-through, essential for the establishment of a new treatment relationship, can be completed only after the change has occurred. The problem is essentially the second therapist's, although the first therapist has to bear the brunt of the child's feelings about the prospective change and also needs to deal with the child's fantasies about the new therapist.

A treatment alliance based on a patient's wish for help may continue during the period of transition. This alliance might be the predominant motive allowing the child to accept the change of therapist in spite of resentment about the change. Despite children's readiness to form new object relationships, as evidenced in their adjustment to new teachers and classmates, there is an important difference in the child's relationship to the therapist in that the analytic work facilitates the development of transference, which makes the relationship to the therapist a very special one for the child.

4

Change of Setting

Various changes in the treatment situation may affect the analytic material of the child patient and cause technical difficulties to arise. There are many different reactions to these changes; the nature or the degree of the reaction depends on the nature of the child's disturbance.

Borderline and severely traumatized children are particularly vulnerable in regard to their feelings of safety and security and therefore may react to any kind of change with massive anxiety. For less severely disturbed children, external changes in the treatment situation may trigger the fear that past traumatic experiences will be repeated. Obsessional children may deal with changes by instituting some form of ritual, such as a particular way of saying "goodbye," but may show anxiety until such defenses are established. Any child may use an external change as a focus for either furthering the analytic work or serving the purposes of resistance.

In the case of Kenny K. there was a reaction to a change of time of appointment. Kenny began treatment at the age of six years three months, and the indexing was done when he was nine years three months old:

It was necessary for the therapist to change one treatment hour per week to 8:00 A.M. instead of the usual after-school session. Kenny wanted all his hours changed to this time because, with the change, he experienced feelings of increased intimacy and of occupying a unique position. At the earlier

To Index: Describe the patient's reactions to unavoidable changes, as of treatment room, appointment times, toys or equipment, therapist's appearance or status (e.g. wearing an engagement or wedding ring, pregnancy, injury), and clinic amenities or auxiliary staff.

hour his father had to bring and return Kenny by car instead of his coming on his own. Moreover, Kenny was the first and only patient in the building at that time.

ANNA FREUD   It is interesting to see what a change of the hour, say to eight o'clock in the morning, done for practical reasons, means to a variety of children. One child may feel, "She only wants me at that time because nobody else would be able to come then." The next child may feel, "I'm very special, I'm allowed to come at eight o'clock." Another child, "I hate to get up in the morning when the whole house is asleep." The next child, "It's nice to get up early when only my father is awake to make my breakfast." There is a whole range of reactions possible.

A change may have quite different meanings for different children, depending on the child's personality and problems, the current material of the analysis, and the link with events in the child's life, which might, for example, suggest that the change was a punishment. Similar considerations arise if a child is seen at a clinic on a Saturday morning, when the clinic is officially closed. Children given appointments for such times seem to feel either very special or discriminated against. A child may not have any special reaction, however, so a therapist should not be too eager to read a particular meaning into the patient's reaction or lack of it.

External changes occur more often in the child analytic setting than in adult analysis. Toys and equipment are changed or modified during the course of treatment. School events, illnesses, and holidays intervene more frequently. In addition, the child experiences his own biological development. In a clinic there are many other activities that impinge on the child; for example, he sees new faces in the corridors. Above all, the child patient interacts with and has direct visual and other contact with the therapist to a much greater degree than the adult analytic patient, who usually uses the couch.

A change of room may have important effects on the child. Some children react by treating such a change as an ordinary occurrence, others as a mild inconvenience, still others as a new experience, and then there are those who are extremely upset by it. Ideally the therapist picks up whatever is helpful for the analytic work, whether the child's response is simply a reaction to reality or involves the child in other ways, as by reviving past traumatic experiences. The length and intensity of the child's response and the repercussions on the psychoanalytic work are important considerations for the therapist, even though all of these effects need not be understood in terms of the current analytic material. Changes may also be occurring because the analytic material has been deflected away from the path of development it previously followed.

A change of place and time of appointment can affect the flow of material, as shown in the case of Oliver U., who began treatment aged six years two months and whose material was indexed when he was eight years ten months old:

> In the eleventh week of treatment there was a change of time at the parents' request, which necessitated also a change of room. Up to this point Oliver's behavior in treatment had been characterized by provocative and controlling enactments. In the new room, Oliver at once brought up material in which both he and the therapist were seen as having been displaced from the previous room and therefore having joined in alliance.

Although the change of room made a profound change in Oliver's previous battle with his analyst, such a change might have occurred in any case once the patient had come to feel that the therapist was an ally. It could also be that the child's anger was redirected toward the parents and that the therapist ceased for a while to be an object of hostile transference because the child had something real to be angry about. Such a reaction is not the same as a defensive displacement of the anger from the therapist onto a convenient external object, in this case the parents. From the child's point of view, he had every reason to be angry with the parents, and his attitude allowed the alliance with the therapist to develop.

Account should also be taken of the fact that the change and its aftermath fitted in with the child's own needs and with the development of his analysis. The experience is an example of how an external change can be used by a child to bring into the analysis his feelings about being "pushed around." A therapist does not introduce such changes intentionally in order to stimulate material, but a child's reactions to inevitable changes can be useful in the analysis. Another child might have blamed the therapist for the change, even if it were instigated by the parents, while still another might have felt humiliated that he was getting a worse room than before.

The therapist has to prepare the child in some way for a change in the treatment room or treatment time, which usually entails explaining the reality involved. With certain patients it is appropriate for a therapist to say, "No one likes changes," or "Lots of people do not like to change," and then to deal with the child's reactions.

It is difficult for some student therapists (and experienced therapists) to prepare the child patient for changes and to explain the reality involved. Students tend to communicate with the child entirely through psychoanalytic "interpretation" rather than through demonstration, in a human way, of their understanding of the child's reaction to unpleasant events such as a change of room. There is a natural tendency for beginning analysts to be frightened of departing from a strictly interpretive stance. Later on it is usually easier to be more natural and human in conversation with patients.

ANNA FREUD   It would be easier if students were not taught the opposite somewhere, usually by their own analyst—because it is natural for human beings to be human. But if their analysts and teachers turn them into something wooden, and then try to turn them back into human beings, it becomes difficult!

If the therapist behaves like a robot and at the first meeting feels he should make contact with the child only by giving "profound" interpretations, he may not win the child's confidence. He may even frighten the child away. For this reason, contact with normal children apart from the analytic experience is essential for the child analyst and should always be a basic training requirement. Without such experience, the therapist's whole approach to a child is in danger of becoming artificial. For example, when asked what she would do if a child sneezed, Anna Freud replied simply, "I would say, 'Have you got a hanky?' "

The "humanity" of the therapist is as much a concern in work with adults as with children. Yet therapists seem at times to advocate a rather cold, aloof, and sterile attitude toward patients, which is probably easier to maintain with adults than with children. There appear to be two extremes of attitude for the child therapist in this area, both of which interfere with the analysis. One extreme is to become rigidly defensive in order to avoid interacting with the patient, and the other is to lose the analytic attitude and become just another "real" person for the patient.

The general rule of therapy is to keep all aspects of the external situation as stable as possible in order to give the internal forces the widest scope for expression. Yet there are no rules spelling out the ideal arrangements for a treatment room and the things to be avoided. There has been much controversy, for example, over whether sand and water should always be provided.

ANNA FREUD   Such questions are based on assumptions which give too great an importance to the external arrangements in the analytic setting. An analyst may do a very bad analysis in what might be considered a perfect treatment room. Another may do a quite effective analysis in a room that has not been devised for a child.

Toys are used in child psychoanalysis to provide a medium of expression for the child because he cannot readily free associate. Sometimes, however, it may be the therapist, and not the child, who needs a new game or toy in order to tolerate the work of the analysis. The principle followed at the clinic is to begin analysis with a certain minimum of toys with which, it is hoped, the particular child will be able to express himself. The toys are not viewed as the tools of the trade; rather the therapist is the main tool. Just as in adult analysis it is left up to the patient to decide what particular mixture of reality, fantasy, and transference he will bring in, so in child analysis it is left up to the child how fully to express his thoughts, fantasies, and wishes directly toward the person of the therapist, how much to use the medium of the toys, and how far to account verbally for experiences at school and at home.

ANNA FREUD   The use of toys cannot be contrasted with the analysis of the transference. It is not one or the other, but one helps the other. That which is really important is what the analyst says and how the analyst and patient relate to each other. The special role of the toy as a therapeutic agent has been greatly overvalued.

Child as well as adult patients often notice aspects of reality associated with the analytic situation but do not report their observations directly. The therapist hopes to pick up this material whether the child verbalizes it indirectly or expresses it in other ways.

ANNA FREUD   Wilhelm Reich, who lived on the second or third floor, once told of a patient in resistance who, when departing, had written on the staircase wall, "The analyst is an ass." Reich found it very useful to notice which of his patients mentioned the inscription in their analyses. Everybody saw it, but with some patients it never turned up in their associations. To a lesser degree, the same sort of process occurs in connection with things which patients observe about their analyst. When such an item appears in an association, perhaps a week later, I usually ask the patient what he has done with it during the week: Where was it? Has he forgotten it? Has he denied it? It must have been quite difficult to carry it around for a week.

It is not only the patient who reacts to changes in the treatment situation. The therapist may also react to changes of various sorts. He may, for example, be exasperated if he finds the treatment room left in a mess by the previous therapist. The patient may react in his turn to the therapist's reaction, but he will tend to do so in a way that reflects his own past. The child who observes his mother's moods extremely closely may react to every little sign of mood change in the therapist. Anna Freud once had an adult patient who was so sensitive that, he said, he could even notice the grass growing! As a child he had been intensely close to his mother, observing every change in her.

The more closely the changes in treatment setting involve the person of the therapist, the more difficult it is for the therapist to sort out which of the patient's reactions reflect transference and which are a natural response to external change. This is not a question of the child's reactions being all one or all the other but, rather, a question of the proportion.

Various aspects of technique involving change are illustrated in the case of Tammy L., who began treatment when she was eleven and was indexed when she was twelve:

The first focus of analytic work was on Tammy's behavioral difficulties as they were linked with her overly close relationship to her mother. After six months, pubertal advances including breast development and menstruation came to the fore, together with conflicts over penis envy and masturbation. With this material Tammy brought transference fantasies about marrying the (female) therapist, finally asking a direct question about whether the therapist had a fiancé. The therapist had wondered for some time how much and in what ways Tammy's material might be influenced by her own marriage plans. On this particular day the therapist felt taken aback by Tammy's question because she had in fact just decided on a wedding date and felt somewhat excited. Shortly afterward there was a long summer vacation, which Tammy anticipated with appropriate sadness. On her return to treatment, Tammy spoke of meeting her first boyfriend during the holidays, but only in the next week did she make a direct reference to the wedding ring which the therapist now wore. Tammy drew a left hand with a line on the wedding finger. At this point the therapist verbalized Tammy's thoughts about her wearing a wedding ring. A completely silent session ensued. Tammy subsequently expressed anxiety over loss of the therapist or the therapist's love in the context of revived oedipal fantasies, and she produced a cover memory of being trapped in a cot as a baby. For the first time Tammy brought fantasies and ideas of intercourse and pregnancy. She later wondered if the therapist were sick (pregnant) and whether she would be seeing a new therapist.

In Tammy's case the therapist used a cautious approach in not introducing material about her own impending marriage. The therapist probably had to counteract her own desire to tell the patient what was happening. Such caution on the therapist's part is well advised. Therapists must become accustomed to keeping their personal preoccupations separated from their patients' material while maintaining an awareness of what is going on in themselves and in the patients.

Another way of handling this situation would have been to interpret Tammy's thoughts and fantasies about penis envy, dating, and marrying the therapist earlier, before these interpretations had reference to the therapist's impending marriage. However, in this case the patient was not only in an early stage of analysis, when such interpretations are not appropriate, but was also in treatment somewhat unwillingly, probably because of her intense involvement with her mother. Moreover, Tammy soon became preoccupied with her pubertal development, so her fantasies could as easily have been connected with her reactions to the physical changes in her own body. Thus Tammy's material might well have followed the same course regardless of the evidence of changes in the therapist's personal life. Even though Tammy had noticed the ring on the therapist's finger and correctly inferred the therapist's marriage, her material might not have been significantly affected by this information because it was following a path of development of its own, linked with her entry into puberty.

A therapist's change in marital status or even a visible pregnancy may not be merely a reality change for the patient. Analytic experience suggests that the therapist's marital state, for example, may be perceived by the patient in a way which is affected by his own fantasies and by the current state of the transference without much reference to reality factors. A child may see a married therapist for a year and even call her Mrs. "X," then one day urgently ask her if she is married. On the other hand, if the child does notice a reality change, it is only natural for him to react to it in some way. This includes, for example, reactions to such things as a change in the therapist's clothes and appearance or hair style. And for the therapist to dress identically each day simply for the sake of minimizing changes in the analytic situation would be a caricature of psychoanalytic technique. A distinction must be maintained between the patient's acknowledgment of reality, his denial or negation of a piece of perceived reality, and his misconstruing of perceptions.

Tammy may have been one of those children affected by an intense closeness to their mother in such a way that they become highly sensitive to the smallest change in the people around them. Sensitivity was, in fact, a characteristic aspect of Tammy's relationships. Her case illustrates the difficulties involved in teasing out the interaction of internal and external factors in the evolution of analytic material. It shows once again that the important element is not the external change in itself, but, rather, how it is used by both the patient and the therapist.

Part Two

The Therapeutic Relationship

5

Treatment Alliance

The treatment alliance is a product of the child's conscious or unconscious wish to cooperate and his readiness to accept the therapist's aid in overcoming internal difficulties and resistances. The alliance is not motivated simply by the child's desire to gain pleasure
from treatment. It involves an acceptance of the need to deal with
internal problems and to do analytic work in the face of internal resistance or external resistance, as from the family. It represents the
coming together of many elements.

In child analysis, as in the analysis of adults, the success of the
analysis may depend upon the patient's attitude toward treatment
and the therapist. The way in which the child uses or attempts to use
the treatment situation and the therapist at different times and under
varying circumstances during the analysis is not an outcome of the
child's transference alone. There are aspects of the child's relationship to the therapist and to treatment which are not transference.
These aspects include elements of the treatment alliance. Although it
is difficult to differentiate clearly between treatment alliance and
transference, a distinction should always be made between the two.

In the treatment alliance, particular motives determine the willingness of the child to work with the therapist at any one time.

ANNA FREUD   The most mature motive is the wish to be assisted in
coping with internal difficulty. Sometimes children really do
express a need for such help, especially children with anxieties

To Index: Describe the steps in the formation of the treatment alliance as it
develops from the child's initial attitudes to therapy. Note any failure in the
development of an adequate treatment alliance and the reasons for it, if known.

and some obsessional children. For example, a borderline child now in treatment is clearly carried in therapy at all times solely by the enormous demand, "Who will help me?" The therapist's role is to relieve the pressure and to be the person who helps him. However, to regard the treatment alliance as based only on the more mature elements, such as a wish for help with internal difficulties, is to oversimplify the situation. Another motive within the general context of the treatment alliance is an aspect of the positive transference: the analyst is the representative of the important adult whose lead is followed, who is trusted and believed as a helping adult, and, as a consequence, with whom the child is willing to work. In other cases the central motive for the alliance might be to please the therapist, who is interested in worries, or the alliance might be based on the child's relationship to the therapist as the mother who tries to understand him. A further motive would be the child's experience of the analyst as a new object of a sort he has never experienced before, a person with a new understanding which in itself arouses positive feelings in the child. The analyst must know at which period in life each motive or attitude belongs, what behavior to expect from the child at each period, and at what age and under what conditions the various factors in the treatment alliance tend to break down. Then, with individual patients, the therapist can observe the steps in the formation of the treatment alliance, on the one hand, and the breakdown of the alliance, on the other.

The child contributes to the therapeutic alliance, as does the therapist; they each make their respective contributions. The treatment alliance also contains components that are neither libidinal nor aggressive, which are linked to the ego or the superego.

ANNA FREUD   In the earlier literature, ego factors were included under the German term *Krankheitseinsicht* (insight into the illness). This was not insight into the factors causing the illness, but insight into the fact of being ill. The term was used with adult patients, referring to the degree that the patient had insight into or awareness of the fact that he was ill. If he had this insight, he would ally himself with somebody in order to do something about it. This was obviously an ego attitude, the ego being conscious of the fact that it was under pressure from various sides and needed help.

Perhaps too sophisticated a demand is placed on young children if therapists ask that they be aware of internal difficulties and that they work with the therapist in order to overcome them. For the young child the positive tie to the therapist probably forms the main basis for the therapeutic work. The older child is expected to develop a proportionately greater awareness of his problems and a greater wish to work toward their solution; for him less of the work should depend on a positive relationship with the therapist.

A distinction should be made between the directly sexual components of positive transference and the so-called aim-inhibited or de-sexualized ones. Such a distinction helps the therapist to see the instinctual, especially the libidinal, components of the treatment alliance, and to separate them from the noninstinctual elements, the ego and superego. The aim-inhibited libidinal elements, which take the form of "liking the therapist," should become a constant factor in the treatment alliance. A child's past experience of a good relationship, as with his mother, can carry over in the relationship to the new object, namely the therapist, as a "background transference" component which can foster a treatment alliance and help to maintain it.

Attachment to treatment is formed on the basis of a wide variety of direct or indirect pleasures or gratifications. If no one at home plays games with a child, for example, he might like to come to treatment because there a grown-up pays attention to him. Such an attachment is distinct from the treatment alliance. The alliance proper should also be distinguished from such aspects of the child's relationship to the therapist as identification with the therapist.

A solid alliance on the basis of a need for understanding and help with internal difficulties is not the same as a positive transference even though positive transference may assist the alliance.

ANNA FREUD   In the past, discussion centered around the general idea of "positive transference." It was thought that, especially at the beginning of a child's analysis, long stretches of the analytic work were made possible by the positive transference. This was an acceptable state of affairs and presented danger in only two respects. The first was the danger that the positive transference could go far beyond what is now called the treatment alliance and could lead to the overwhelming wish to live out in reality the love for the analyst. The second was the risk that, with the change from a positive to a negative transference, the patient's cooperation with the analyst could break down.

If the analysis depends for its existence only on the maintenance of positive transference, then it may be limited in what it can achieve and perhaps also in its duration. Moreover, not all positive transference contributes to or assists a treatment alliance. For example, a sexualized positive transference may work against a successful alliance, in that the patient's wish for a particular type of "working together" may run counter to the progress of therapy.

In practice, the state of the transference always has repercussions on the treatment alliance, and the alliance is not completely autonomous and independent of the transference, even though a conceptual distinction is made between treatment alliance and transference. The "honeymoon period" in analysis, for example, may be based to a large extent on an initial positive transference.

A certain confusion exists in the use of the terms "positive" and "negative" transference. Negative transference is sometimes but not always a resistance. It might be a manifestation of resistance, for example to the development of positive, loving feelings, but it might also be the transfer of hostile feelings from an original object toward the person of the therapist and thus part of the developing analytic material. Similarly, positive transference is sometimes a manifestation of resistance. Although positive transference may represent affectionate feelings toward the therapist, it may also be a mode of resisting the expression of underlying hostile and resentful attitudes.

The treatment alliance also relies on the patient's feelings of trust, on the pleasure to be obtained from talking to someone, and on the satisfaction gained from the therapeutic work, all of which reinforce the patient's cooperation. A warm and positive feeling toward the therapist also arises because of the therapist's contribution in being able to understand and put into words something that has bothered the patient, and this feeling too is not transference proper. The therapist is liked for having helped.

ANNA FREUD   The analyst is a new and understanding object, different from the former objects. The patient forms a positive tie to the
analyst on the basis of this difference, and the tie can be viewed as
transference only in a sense so broad that every tie is seen as
transference. The patient's ego seeks an ally to overcome internal
difficulties.

From the side of the child a contribution to the treatment alliance
comes from the child's conscience. The superego causes the child to
feel that he ought to come to therapy even if he does not wish to or is
not in the mood. The normal role of the conscience in the treatment
alliance becomes obvious when guilt feelings about missed sessions
are absent and the patient turns to sources of gratification outside the
therapeutic setting, allowing himself to miss sessions in order to do
so. The patient's superego, it might be said, has not insisted on his
attending the session.

The role of the superego element in the treatment alliance is illustrated by the treatment of Quentin J., who began treatment at the age
of nine years one month and who was thirteen years five months
when the indexing was done:

Quentin's attendance was irregular and he did not seem to have a very
strong wish to get better. He clung to his symptom of enuresis and enjoyed
the secondary gain of having mother interested in his body functions. His
"weak" superego allowed him to be unconcerned over the matter of missed
sessions, and a proper treatment alliance was not established. This was particularly so in the first half of the second year, at which time Quentin missed
one session nearly every week, without any sign of guilt. He gave no previous warning, and the missed session was always to gratify some impulse. He
would go home after school to have a snack and watch television or sometimes to go to the lavatory, or he missed the session because he had "been
mucking about"—Quentin's euphemism for a number of pleasurable activities on a primitive or fantasy level. If the parents did not take active responsibility, Quentin just drifted.

The commitment to attend sessions, even when strong resistance
is present, can play a part in the global, broad, and descriptive sense
of the treatment alliance. The question of the extent to which a
therapist should express criticism or disapproval to the child in regard to "unnecessarily" missed sessions is a difficult one, as the
therapist may unwittingly be drawn into a sadomasochistic relation-

ship with the patient or may find herself unconsciously responding to a transference role which the child is attempting to induce in her. By not coming to sessions, the child may attempt to provoke the therapist and force her to act as a superego or as a critical parent; missing a session is not then simply a resistance or acting out. The therapist must monitor her countertransference, making use of it as far as possible for greater understanding of her patient.

As for the contributions made by the therapist to the treatment alliance, early in therapy the therapist's tasks include finding some way to help the child become aware of a painful internal situation or conflict. The therapist may help to develop in the child a wish to find relief through treatment. For the wish to develop, however, there must first be in the child a capacity for self-observation and some awareness that there is an internal problem.

The child does not often feel his symptoms to be painful. Rather, the parents or others in the child's life feel the pain and make the child come for treatment; in this way they participate in the treatment alliance. The notion of a treatment alliance can be linked with the therapist's awareness that the patient is feeling pain or discomfort, so that the therapist understands her task as that of helping the child as a patient to develop the treatment alliance. In the case of a child with temper tantrums, for example, although it is others who suffer because of the tantrums, the development of the child's wish to be helped to deal with an internal painful problem depends on the therapist helping him to become aware that what precedes or causes the tantrums lies mainly within himself, rather than in the external environment.

With adolescent patients their positive attachment to the object and their wish for help with internal problems are not always sufficient to carry the therapeutic work through in the face of the mistrust, suspicion, skepticism, and doubt that they so often experience in association with their efforts to break the ties with the parental figure.

ANNA FREUD   With adults the problem is much simpler, because if the treatment alliance sinks below a specific level, the patient stops treatment. However, if in spite of professed unwillingness and absence of treatment alliance, the patient still comes, the analyst may suspect rightly that something else holds him in treatment, and the analyst is apt to try to find out what it is. Is it a libidinal element, or is it a treatment alliance which he covers up? But with the child, all this is obscured by the fact that coming is not of his own volition. In fact, what the analyst says to the parents is, "It is part of your task to help the child come at times when he does not want to come." The analyst recognizes that the child is very much more apt to break the treatment alliance, because the mature part of him that holds him in analysis during phases of negative transference and resistance is less developed.

When a positive alliance exists between the analyst and parents, they tend to bring the child to treatment when he will not or cannot overcome his resistance on his own—that is, when the treatment alliance between child and therapist is absent or weak. At times a degree of parental pressure is necessary in such cases. It is the parents who must have the determination to carry on with treatment in spite of counterforces. Naturally parents vary in the ways in which they bring pressure to bear on the child. Some try to persuade the child, to show him that attendance at treatment is important for him and them. Others bribe the child. Still others actually drag the child to treatment.

Difficulties are placed in the path of the analytic work when there is no alliance with the parents, or when there is a "negative" alliance, which may even interfere with the child's attendance at therapy. This can happen, for example, when the parents are jealous of the child's affection for the therapist. The parents may subtly oppose the child's wish to come to treatment or may collude with his resistance. Often the way in which the child brings up material and behaves toward the therapist in the analysis reflects the attitudes of his parents to his treatment.

The therapist should actively work to encourage the treatment alliance. It is crucial, for example, that the therapist verbalize for the child the child's anxieties about treatment and attempt to reduce them to more manageable proportions as early in the treatment as possible. Doing so helps the child to see that the therapist's role is not only that of a sympathetic listener but in addition that of a person who can understand and, through this understanding, be of help. The verbalization of anxieties and frightening fantasies about treatment is not necessarily the same as interpreting the transference though the therapist's comments may refer to the child's thoughts about the therapist's person.

The treatment alliance is strengthened by efforts of the therapist to make the treatment situation attractive to the child, and these can to some extent counterbalance the resistance. The therapy should not be all hard work for the patient.

ANNA FREUD   The analyst's goal is to maintain the patient's willingness to work together at a level which will make it possible to deal
with whatever comes up. There are moments when the analyst
may interrupt the analytic work to say, "I think we have worked
hard enough at that today; let's play a little now." It is important
not to put too much pressure on the child, or to raise the child's
anxiety too high. It has to be kept at a level which the child is
willing to endure.

Facilitating the child's entry into analytic treatment by sustaining a certain level of attractiveness of the treatment differs significantly from "seducing" the child by offering gratifications unrelated to the analytic work. On learning that some people mistakenly believed that child analysts at Hampstead gave children sweets in the treatment sessions, Anna Freud remarked, "You can tell them that the Hampstead children bring their own sweets."

When child analysis was in its infancy, it was thought necessary to have a preparatory phase before the analysis proper could begin.

ANNA FREUD   The preparatory phase notion was instituted for reasons which different analysts understood in different ways. Some
analysts understood it as an intensification and deliberate arousal
of the positive transference to the new person (the analyst), which
then made a treatment alliance possible. People like August Aichhorn and me, for example, had in mind drawing the child's attention to the internal conflict, arousing the child's own hostility toward the pathological part in himself, and then basing the
treatment alliance on that. Aichhorn may be misunderstood as
having as his main intention the wish to show the patient that the
therapist is not hostile and that he is on the side of the child. But
his main intention actually was to create an inner "split" in the
patient and then to base the treatment on that split. His technique

of "outdoing" the delinquent by telling stories of his own youthful delinquency was for the purpose of establishing a new identification which could lead to the inner split.

Some children who appear to have little insight into their problems nevertheless develop from the beginning an extremely friendly attitude toward the therapist. In instances where the child immediately forms a strong positive attachment, the question arises how much this is based on object hunger—consequent, for example, on early deprivation—and how much on a character transference of some kind, on a habitual mode of relating. Such quickly formed relationships may also serve defensive functions. Although an immediate, almost ready made affectionate relationship is not a proper treatment alliance, it may, while it lasts, be useful for therapeutic work.

The child's cooperation with the therapist depends on the presence of a wish in the child to communicate some of his problems and anxieties. The relative absence of such a wish, or the presence of a strong need to defend against communication, and the effect of this absence on the treatment alliance, was evident in the case of a girl who would not discuss anything with the therapist. She wrote in a diary during the session and kept another private diary at home in which she wrote very different things. The danger she felt to be inherent in communicating was so great for this child that, after letting the analyst know that she had the private diary, she stopped writing in it, and it was never possible to establish an adequate treatment alliance.

There are at least two definitions of treatment alliance. The first is a broad descriptive umbrella, a composite of all those factors that keep the patient in treatment and which enable him to remain there during phases of resistance and hostile transference. The second is a narrower definition based specifically on the patient's awareness of illness and on his feeling of a need to do something about it, linked with the presence in him of a capacity to tolerate the effort and pain of facing internal conflict. In line with the wider definition, the therapeutic relationship can, for a time, be maintained predominantly on the basis of gratifications containing instinctual elements, such as love for the analyst or object hunger. Such aspects are the id elements in the therapeutic alliance. At other times the treatment relationship appears to be based more on the ego elements included in the narrower definition. Ideally, the therapist should attempt to be sensitive to the different ingredients of the treatment alliance at any particular time, as the alliance fluctuates in strength, composition, and stability.

For a variety of reasons a treatment alliance sometimes fails to develop.

ANNA FREUD   I had a young adolescent girl in treatment. She was unwilling to be in analysis, and there was a complete absence of a treatment alliance. Her previous analyst had tried to attack the problem for two years by interpretation, with no result. I tried to deal with the problem by circumventing it, also with no positive result as far as the treatment alliance was concerned. I would not say there were no changes in symptoms, but the absence of a treatment alliance remained absolutely firm. There was no phobic attitude, but the patient had made a decision to keep her private life private: no one had the right to intrude. When she had an excess of examination anxiety and was told how much her parents wanted to help, her answer was, "I wish they'd leave me in peace," which meant, "I wish they'd leave it to me." Her adamant answer to interpretations of that attitude was, "I prefer people who keep their private affairs private," probably based on a masturbation conflict which had to be kept secret. I did not think there was a complete absence of insight into inner difficulties, but there was the conviction that inner difficulties have to be combated by being strict with oneself. This is an extreme, almost fossilized strictness of character structure. How to create a treatment alliance was beyond me.

In another case, an adolescent boy who had no treatment alliance nevertheless improved as a result of treatment. The idea of "getting better" thus omits the distinction between the aim of gaining symptom relief and that of restoring the child, through therapy, to the path of normal development. The question arises whether this boy had merely experienced an improvement in his symptoms or had in fact been analyzed.

ANNA FREUD   I would say it was an analysis in the case of this boy. I know that his sense of masculinity was restored as a consequence of the analytic work done on his aggression and inhibitions. Transference feelings were intense, but what was transferred was not in itself helpful to the analytic work. He never had a treatment alliance, and the therapist worked continually for the establishment of an alliance, in the sense that he might feel, "I really need to change, and you are the person to help me to change." The patient reluctantly let himself be dragged through the analysis, essentially on the basis of his passivity, which might have contained masochistic or homosexual elements. It was as though he said, "If you want me to get somewhere, drag me there."

Such behavior can be viewed as "treatment compliance" rather than treatment alliance. In another clinical example, therapy was a constant struggle in which treatment was eventually broken off. Esther L., who began treatment at the age of eight years ten months, was indexed when she was nine years eleven months:

When Esther began treatment, she reacted with extreme anxiety. Her mother reported that she was unwilling to come, and Esther even went to the length of hiding in a disused building when it was time to leave home for the clinic. Yet the extreme nature of this reaction would not have been known without the mother's description, as it was not apparent to the analyst in Esther's sessions. Although she was rather silent, her movements were restricted, and she kept busy with modeling and drawing, she came with her therapist from the waiting room to the treatment room quite readily and seemed reasonably friendly. Her initial anxiety was reduced by interpretations of her thoughts and feelings about treatment, in particular her fear that the therapist might tell tales about her to her parents and her belief that she had been brought to the clinic as a punishment because her parents felt there was something wrong with her. For some time, however, she continued to view the treatment as punishment. Following the first vacation break, after eleven weeks of treatment, she did not want to return to treatment and screamed and cried, begging her mother not to make her come. She told her mother that she was sent to treatment as punishment for wanting to hurt her sister, and she promised to be "good" in future.

There is a variety of possible reasons for such a "basic unwillingness" to enter treatment (as opposed to a resistance to treatment). These include the existence of family secrets, loyalty conflicts, and deep-seated disturbances in object relationships. A child's basic unwillingness may also express the unconscious ambivalence of one or both parents about the child's receiving treatment. This is particularly the case when there are family secrets, or when the disturbance in the child is so tied to a disturbance in one of the parents that an unconscious collusion between parent and child is threatened by the treatment.

In addition, an unwillingness to enter treatment often derives from mistrust, which in many cases appears to be a defense against the formation of a positive attachment. This defensive posture may at times be motivated by an expectation of being "dropped," of being disappointed or rejected. What is called mistrust is not necessarily a basic disturbance in object relationships. It is a characteristic trait, for example, of adolescence. In contrast to this sort of mistrust, typical of a particular developmental phase, there is another type of basic mistrust which is transferred from an earlier object relationship. In such cases the development of a positive transference does not take place in a way that permits analytic work to evolve, and a trusting relationship may take years to be established, or may never occur. A basic mistrust might also be present from the very earliest months of life, and the therapist might thus be confronted with a form of character transference. But when the mistrust develops relatively late and there are also positive features to the child's object attachments, a trusting relationship to the therapist may develop in time.

Another reason for unwillingness to enter treatment is the fact that for certain children therapy is tedious work or provides insufficient pleasurable gain. A great deal depends on the skill of the therapist in being able to arouse the child's interest in facing the therapeutic task. From a descriptive point of view, all these situations might be called resistances to treatment, but they are not all equally amenable to interpretation.

Finally, there are those puzzling cases when children continue to come to sessions even though it is not at all apparent why. Nothing seems to happen in the session, and the therapist appears to make little or no contribution; yet the patient improves. Whereas what the therapist does or does not do may not be important for these children, her presence as a therapist and her personal characteristics may be of more therapeutic importance than is generally realized.

6

Resistance

It has been said that psychoanalysis consists essentially of the analysis of the patient's resistances to free association. This cannot be the case in child analysis since free association does not play the same role there as it does in the analysis of adults. The child analytic setting provides many different ways in which analytically significant material can be expressed, and one of the initial tasks of the therapist is to enable the child to provide material in a suitable way. But however suitable the analytic setting provided by the therapist, resistances to the analysis inevitably develop.

Resistance differs from a basic unwillingness of the child to participate in the analytic process, in which case the child has no real wish for treatment. Resistances develop during the course of treatment as a consequence of the analytic process. They are related to such factors as transference development and the operation of defenses against the emergence of anxiety-evoking material.

In child analysis it is necessary to look for resistances to communication or to cooperation in general rather than resistances to verbal free association in particular. The very concept of resistance is difficult to define in relation to child pychoanalysis.

ANNA FREUD   Resistances may be more difficult to detect in child analysis than in adult analysis. With adults, analysts know that a

To Index: Indicate the frequency, intensity, and duration of resistance, along with variations in its form, pattern, or content. Note significant links between specific content and resistance, as well as the role and use of external factors (e.g., parental attitudes) by the child for the purposes of resistance. Comment on changes in resistance, as well as in the therapist's method of dealing with them, whether successful or not.

resistance has occurred when the process of free association is interfered with in some way. Since there is no free association in child analysis, analysts have much greater difficulty in detecting the indications of resistance and knowing how and when a child is "in resistance."

Some resistances are present from the beginning of treatment and are inherent in the mental structure of the patient. These may be called "character resistances." As with adults, there is a type of juvenile patient who does not allow anxiety to find expression in thought or words but constantly negates it. Some resistances (using the term broadly and descriptively) start to operate with the very idea of coming to analysis. These must be distinguished from a basic unwillingness to undergo treatment and also from the specific resistances that arise during the course of analysis and which are related to the material the child brings up. It is important to differentiate between the type of resistance shown and the particular content that is being defended against.

The psychic structure of the child and the particular way in which he communicates at any particular stage in his development can modify the way in which resistances are manifested, their form, and the content against which they operate. An illustration of resistance comes from the case of Dorothy J., who was indexed at five years five months of age, after one year eight months of treatment:

At times Dorothy fought against unwelcome interpretations by the therapist, uttering such typical protests as "Shut up," "Stop talking," or putting her fingers in her ears and saying, "I can't hear you." Two specific phrases indicating her resistance—"I'm not taking any notice of you" and "Mind your own business"—derived from what she had heard during family quarrels.

When a child behaves like Dorothy, it may be that the reaction is stimulated by the degree of anxiety stirred up by the therapist's interpretations. However, the child may in fact accept what the therapist is saying but convey by her action or response that she cannot take any more at that point. Her resistance may be to the analytic procedure at that stage rather than to the content of the interpretation.

Common to all resistances is the patient's holding something back or unconsciously wanting to shut something out of awareness.

ANNA FREUD   Even in analysis of adults resistance is not simply resistance to free association. Although early in the history of analysis resistance was most easily detected in regard to disturbances in
the flow of free associations, resistance is in fact any interruption
of the analytic process brought about by the patient which occurs
despite the willingness of the patient to undergo the analysis.
However, when free association begins to be interrupted, a resistance is occurring which needs to be analyzed. When someone
says that there is something on his mind but he cannot quite put
his finger on it, and then tries to say what comes into his mind, he
is working against the defenses which result in a resistance. He
can either overcome that resistance with an inner effort or be
helped by the analyst to overcome it by interpretation. But that is
merely the connection between defense and resistance. To view
the resistances as a clinical manifestation of the functioning of the
mechanisms of defense, as what has been called "ego resistance,"
is to look at one side only. But every defense that the analytic process meets usually reveals itself, in the adult, by a stiffening of the
resistance. Otherwise the defense would not be doing its duty. To
the degree that there is internal conflict, there must always be a
degree of resistance directed against the analytic process.

As a consequence of internal factors, there is always a degree of
resistance against the analytic work, a resistance which is to some
extent counteracted by acceptance of the therapeutic contract or by
the treatment alliance. At certain times, that resistance can increase
in intensity sufficiently to disrupt the normal workings of the analysis. What the analyst labels "resistance" does not necessarily come
into being in the analysis *de novo*.

ANNA FREUD   The analytic process, which aims at uncovering that
which is unconscious, runs counter to the whole structure of the
personality and especially counter to maintaining the individual's
narcissism and the boundary between the repressed and that
which is conscious. Naturally, at a particular point of advance,
equally important resistances against that advance occur.

The flow of analytic material stops or deviates when it meets a resistance, and normally it unfolds a little more following the inter-

pretation of the resistance. In the usual course of events, a further resistance then occurs, which can also be interpreted. It would not be entirely correct, however, to define resistance solely in terms of the unfolding of the patient's material. The process of flow depends on the process of dealing with the resistances, which cannot be done before they have occurred. It is essential for the analyst to spot the resistance early, in *statu nascendi*, before it has grown to such dimensions that the analysis is broken off or reaches a stalemate.

ANNA FREUD   Very often the adult patient says, "I really didn't feel like coming today; I don't know why." This means he has felt a resistance, but it was not so strong that he could not overcome it. In the same circumstances, children may refuse to come. Analysts can help by anticipating resistance, by saying, for example, "Now be very careful after our talk today. You may say to yourself, 'I won't go to that person again,' or 'It's really much too nice a day to come to analysis,' or 'I have so much homework I'd better not come.' " Analysts often anticipate resistance, especially in patients with strong guilt feelings who have opened up and talked about forbidden matters. To such patients, the analyst appears to have been in the role of the seducer and has to be avoided the next day. In general, analysts have to expect an alternation between the unfolding of material and difficulties in the way of that unfolding.

Interpretations "in advance" may be used to warn the patient that he might feel guilty because of the things spoken of or discovered in a particular session. The intention in giving such an interpretation is to help the patient, should he feel himself in resistance, make the decision to come to the next session rather than staying away and to enable him to bring up the material at that session in an accessible way. The patient might say to himself, "If I stayed away now, it would obviously be as anticipated; therefore I had better go," or "I would stay away, but I know that my therapist would say I didn't want to come."

The form of resistance may be significantly linked with the character and personality of the child, and also with his psychopathology. The analyst must determine the form of the patient's resistance, whether it is a massive blocking-out, a subtle intellectualizing, or some other type.

The therapist may frame his interpretation in such a way that it is maximally acceptable to the patient or minimizes resistances which might be aroused by the interpretation. Taking care to do so may aid children, like Dorothy J., who respond to interpretations by such behavior as becoming mute or blocking their ears and yet show, in the flow of material in following sessions, that the interpretation has nonetheless been accepted.

In certain instances the child may find it necessary to appear to reject the interpretation in order to preserve his self-esteem but may nonetheless be able to accept it because it relieves anxiety or guilt. Dorothy's reaction to the interpretation, for example, seems like a resistance but dynamically is probably not. In other instances, the child may appear to accept the interpretation, but nothing happens—no analytic movement occurs. The resistance is hidden from the therapist, who notices it later only because of the lack of analytic progress.

7

Fantasies and Expectations

The child's fantasies, expectations, and beliefs about treatment are greatly influenced by his theories of the world, which are in turn connected with his level of development. He enters treatment with a host of expectations, wishes, fears, beliefs, and theories—some conscious, others unconscious. His beliefs and fantasies affect his attitude to treatment profoundly, leading, for example, to a "positive" attitude to treatment based on the patient's expectation of obtaining direct gratification from it. Equally, he may show a negative attitude to analysis, arising from unverbalized fears and anxieties.

The therapist often must comment on the child's thoughts or expectations even in the very first session. An appropriate interpretation in a first session might involve a child's fears of what will happen to him in treatment. The child's fears in such circumstances are not a manifestation of transference, though many analysts label them as such.

In fact, none of the child's early thoughts about the therapist are inevitably or necessarily transferences, and thus in interpreting or verbalizing them, the therapist is not necessarily interpreting transference. Some therapists consider all thoughts about the therapist to be transference and consequently avoid interpreting them early in treatment, but this reflects bad technique. It is more important to know what is going on, as far as possible, in the mind of the child and to put his thoughts into words if such verbalization assists the analytic process.

To Index: Detail the content of the child's initial fantasies, how they are dealt with, and their fate later in treatment (e.g., their disappearance from the material or their reappearance within the context of the transference). Note the effect of the parents' comments or attitudes.

There are great differences in the degree to which different therapists verbalize the child's initial thoughts about treatment. In the first session some therapists probe for and try to verbalize the child's fears, saying, "You must have thought such and such when you were coming here and feared that such and such would happen to you." Others wait until the child shows signs of anxiety which might interfere with the continuity of treatment. The way the therapist verbalizes the child's initial thoughts about treatment contributes to the analytic climate within which transference interpretations come to be made.

Although the therapist may quickly understand some of the patient's preoccupations, it is not always to the advantage of the analysis to interpret this understanding immediately to the patient. Usually the fantasies and thoughts brought in the first session or two are later understood by the therapist differently, and sometimes more comprehensively. In the beginning, at least, the anxieties of the patient and the resistances with which she comes to analysis should be the focus of interpretation.

ANNA FREUD   What analysts mean by fantasies and expectations about treatment is what the child brings with him into treatment before the transference ever begins. These are therefore not produced by the transference, but they color the transference. The fantasies differ in their effects on the establishment of the treatment alliance. The fantasy that one is a big person if one has analysis is an expectation which means at first that analysis is a nice thing. The expectation that one who is in analysis is crazy is a fantasy that works against the treatment alliance. What the analyst is after is the contrast between what the child brings to the situation and what he then experiences in the situation.

In some children the analysis never really begins because the therapist has failed from the beginning to notice and interpret anxieties and expectations which the child presents in regard to the treatment situation. The therapist should listen very carefully for indications of the child's initial preoccupations and fantasies about treatment. There is always a level of resistance present, and the child's initial fantasies and expectations about treatment may actually be part of his resistance to the analytic process itself. This situation differs from that which may occur later when resistances arise as reactions to the analytic process. Fantasies and expectations about treatment are not in themselves resistances to the analysis, although they may contribute to it, and certainly they are not to be equated with the transference resistances which normally arise during the course of analysis.

The analyst's initial contacts with the child may stimulate and shape his fantasies and expectations in regard to the treatment situation. Concentration camp children treated after the Second World War came to sessions prepared to spend an hour alone with another person, anticipating a highly gratifying experience not available to them elsewhere. In certain circumstances the analytic situation can fulfill the child's wish for an intimate relationship, which contributes to the establishment of a treatment alliance; in other cases the wish can serve as a resistance.

ANNA FREUD   Practically all children derive some pleasure from the daily contact with the analyst. It is the ungratifiable fantasy expectations which interfere more with the analytic process. There are fantasy expectations which cannot find fulfillment in the analytic situation, such as being turned into a boy, having a baby, or becoming the most important person to the analyst or the family.

Development of a transference distortion of an initial set of thoughts about the analysis is common. Transference may make use of the fantasies, thoughts, and wishes with which the child enters analysis. Even the child who initially finds his needs gratified by the toys available in the treatment room or by having an adult to himself for an hour usually begins to establish a transference and to bring useful analytic material. Although real gratifications may persist, other gratifications brought about by the analytic work, such as the relief of anxiety and the pleasure of progressive development, are of quite a different order, and become the significant motivating factors in the analysis.

The clinical example of Helen S. illustrates the effect on a child's initial expectations of what she had been told about treatment. The child began treatment at the age of six years five months; the indexing was done when she was seven years nine months old:

When Helen, a deprived child, started analysis, she thought she was coming to a "club." This idea was given to her by her foster mother, who at the diagnostic stage, against the psychiatrist's advice, described the clinic as a club because she "did not want the child to be worried." Helen's positive attachment to the therapist and to the clinic was noted right away. Throughout the second session she kept repeating that she liked coming and she pleaded for more time. This became a feature in the transference up to the time Helen was withdrawn by the foster mother from treatment.

ANNA FREUD   The case of Helen S. shows how incorrect information can lead to expectations and fantasies about treatment which might conceivably be a hindrance to it. But it is possible to overestimate this factor. Thus, even if the foster mother had not given the child the information she did, it would have emerged very quickly that Helen had an enormous deficit in mothering and was looking for an attentive mother in the analysis. If she had received more mothering at home, she might have been more amenable to treatment. I am reminded of the concentration camp children and of the children from institutions who come to analysis with a need to find an adult who can take the missing mother's place. In a broad sense Helen's response can be called a transference, but what is transferred is the need, the overriding wish which has never been fulfilled in her life—the wish to be mothered. She begs, "Let me stay longer. My foster mother doesn't mind if I don't come home; she would like to get rid of me." All of this may be completely true.

Such strong needs at the beginning of treatment can interfere with the development of a treatment alliance. Helen was brought under false pretenses. Being told, not that she was entering treatment, but that she was joining a club conveyed to her that she was going to have a nice time, which linked with her denial that she had a problem and with her need to have someone be a good mother to her.

Parents like Helen's have dealt with their children for a long time in the same way in similar situations. Their deceptions are connected with a long-standing, mutually defensive situation between child and parent, and if the therapist were to contradict the mother, the child might simply say, "I prefer to believe my mommy, and I don't believe you."

Many other influences affect initial fantasies and expectations of treatment. The analysis of many pairs of siblings shows that children can come with the most peculiar expectations about treatment, based, for example, on their theories about what happened to their siblings during treatment. This happens in spite of their having received a proper preparation by the parents. For Quentin J. who was nine years one month old when treatment began and ten years four months when his case was indexed, the initial fantasies and expectations were influenced by the fact that a brother had been in treatment for some time:

Quentin had a fantasy of treatment as a form of sexual play, derived from his brother's description of what went on in his sessions. To Quentin, whose brother was a borderline psychotic, receiving treatment meant being crazy. In addition to arousing these anxieties, the prospect of undergoing treatment was gratifying to Quentin because it raised his status in the family and gave him what he felt his brother had been given earlier.

The child's early thoughts about analysis may be dispelled within a few days, and the clinical picture change markedly. In other cases, some of the initial fantasies may remain for a long time, reappearing later in different forms in the material. The initial fantasies may come to be linked with subsequent transference development, in which case they may have predictive value as precursors of later transference manifestations.

Material from children's cases shows clearly how the child's own fantasies, on the one hand, and bits and pieces of information derived from the parents, on the other, fuse to determine the child's fantasies and expectations about treatment. One or the other aspect may predominate, depending on the child's current level of development, his preoccupations, needs, wishes, and his past history. It is not always of great clinical importance to discover the source of the child's fantasies and expectations, but it is of extreme importance to put into words, as far as possible, what they are.

8

Insight and Self-Observation

The role of insight as a therapeutic agent is much clearer in adult than in child analysis. Yet insight plays a special part in bringing about changes during the course of analysis, even though it is not the only factor in producing therapeutic change. Curiously, experience with adult patients who were analyzed in childhood shows that they remember of their child analyses only isolated fragments, the significance of which they often do not understand. The therapist may well wonder what has happened to the insight gained in the first analysis, which was considered therapeutically successful. Here the development of insight should be distinguished from other therapeutic changes which have the effect of restoring the child to the path of normal development.

Insight has to do with being in touch with one's feelings, motivations, and behavior, which is possible, of course, without analysis. Insight of this kind, being in touch with one's feelings without necessarily reasoning about and verbalizing the cause of the feelings, may be nearer to a child's analytic experience than to an adult's. The development of insight depends upon a degree of self-observation. It is not possible to have insight without self-observation, but it is possible to have self-observation without insight. Because there is a cognitive element in insight, the child's level of conceptual and intellectual functioning affects his view of the world, including his view of himself and his feelings.

To Index: Illustrate the child's degree of awareness and verbalization of his motives, feelings, wishes, and conflicts. Distinguish development of insight from changes in the child's behavior, attitudes, relationships, and symptoms owing to other causes. Note and illustrate significant changes and fluctuations in insight during the analysis.

Psychoanalysis is not the only way of coming to possess the kind of self-knowledge called "insight," and with or without analysis, people vary tremendously in this ability. Perhaps the early upbringing of the child, especially the manner in which the parents help the child to deal with her feelings, influences and facilitates this kind of insight. If from a very early age a child is told every time she hits another child, "I know you are angry, but it hurts Tommy if you hit him on the head, so don't do it," she may develop a more "useful" piece of insight than the child who is merely told, "That's bad, don't do it." The second approach forces the child to identify with moral authority in a way that is not as insightful. As a consequence, a greater distance may develop between her conscious awareness and her real wishes or feelings, so that she may have no idea about them and hence no insight into them.

ANNA FREUD   The first method of upbringing, which deals with feelings, brings an earlier maturing of the ego. This links with Anny Katan's view about the role of verbalization in early childhood. Verbalization facilitates the maturing of the ego and the acquisition of the capacity for self-observation. The young child tends to externalize his internalized conflicts and then to experience them as a battle between himself and the outside world rather than to see the conflicts as an inner battle. Analysis establishes a consciousness of the inner battle. Long ago, in one of my first cases, an obsessional girl of six complained, "Before I came to analysis, I was just angry, but now since I am with you, I am angry that I am angry, and that's much worse." She had realized what was going on in her, but this was not insight. There is a split in the ego, dividing it into a part that experiences and another part that observes, as Richard Sterba has described. The observing part develops later. When a split like this seems to be present in early childhood, it is in fact a symptom of the obsessional character formation or the obsessional symptomatology of the child.

Children in analysis sometimes report insights and self-observations that are connected with what they have been discussing in the analysis even though the children do not show obsessional precocity.

ANNA FREUD   There is a difference between the development of insight during the analytic process and the sort of obsessional precocity that sometimes appears as part of a normal developmental process. An example of such precocity is the six-year-old child who not only becomes angry but also says, "Look how angry I am at the moment."

Insight is not simply self-observation, nor is it restricted to the so-called "insight into illness" (awareness of illness). Rather, insight has much to do with becoming aware of what has previously been unconscious. Such insight may be gathered in a variety of ways, one of which is through the analytic process.

ANNA FREUD   Self-observation and awareness of what goes on are capacities normal to the mature ego. Analysts try to help the patient make use of these capacities and extend them into the unconscious area of the mind. Patients exhibit these capacities to varying degrees. In some people they are conspicuously absent, in others very little developed, and in still others developed to a high degree. There is a question as to when these capacities come into being. If a child should say, "Every time I hurt myself I get angry with my mother," I would think that she had an unusual piece of insight, namely that bodily hurt creates anger toward an object. But it would not be surprising if a grown man were aware that every time he has an upset day, he gets terribly impatient with his children or his wife. This is not unusual. Such awareness is not expected in the young child, but analysis can make these connections even for the very young.

The child is at first extremely egocentric, and his observations are primarily concerned with his own position in his world. Self-observation is thus, at first, more important to him than observation of and empathy with others. Understanding of or insight into motivations comes relatively late in development and is facilitated for the analytic patient by the treatment process.

ANNA FREUD   The products of early self-observation are externalized immediately in the child. This is something that also occurs in later life, with people who have a particularly low degree of self-observation and self-awareness and are overcritical toward others and not at all critical of themselves.

Self-observation, self-awareness, and insight, though related, differ in the extent to which the unconscious motivations have become part of conscious awareness. Insight refers to a kind of turning to observe oneself, as if to say, "Behind this that I see there must be something else going on." Insight reflects not only a split in the ego but also a development of the superego, which comes to utilize the self-observing function of the ego.

Analytic therapies are distinguished from play therapies in that interpretation, insight, and the self-awareness consequent on interpretation are the major therapeutic agents. Analysts at the Hampstead Clinic do not agree with the idea that analysis provides a corrective or counteracting emotional experience in the sense that the child can "start again," replacing the past with a new relationship experienced with the therapist.

ANNA FREUD   Analysis is neither abreaction, which would be associated with play therapy, nor "corrective emotional experience," as Franz Alexander called it. It is rather the changing of the inner balance or focus to bring about that widening of consciousness which is insight into motivation. These are three different concepts of the therapeutic process. Insight does not occur without a working-through process.

Analysis works by processes that widen the areas of self-observation and consciousness. The widening comes about because both inner resistances and the motives for defending against impulses of one sort or another are reduced. The therapist may indicate, for example, that it is natural to feel angry with mommy or with daddy. As a result, the next time the child talks or even thinks about her parents, she may have less resistance to such thoughts and her conflicts may be more accessible to analysis.

When the child does not have sufficient self-observing capacity, the therapist "lends" it to her in the analytic session. This exchange applies particularly to the very young patient, of age two or three. In children who have a low degree of self-observing capacity, there is less of an ability to continue analytic work outside the session. Since the capacity for self-observation in such children depends so much on the presence of the therapist, they have a special need for frequent sessions to keep therapy effective. Children in general, as compared with adults, have less capacity for self-observation. They also have a greater tendency to externalize. However, in children, as in adults, the self-observing function, whether "borrowed" or not, can at times be used in the service of defense. The child's tendency to externalize and rationalize may reduce his motivation to make use of self-observation.

ANNA FREUD   In other cases self-observation is excessive. There are children (for example, some obsessional children), just as there are similar adults, who are constantly plagued by the feeling that they can "see" themselves. They watch themselves doing whatever it is they are doing, and this gives them a feeling of "unreality." The experience can occur in individuals who are not severely ill. Or there is the insight that some psychotics have, which makes them aware of motivations in others that are usually kept unconscious and repressed. This knowledge on their part has no therapeutic effect on them at all, and the knowledge gained from this sort of insight may even hinder recovery.

A phenomenon in adult patients, not reported with children, is that of self-torture, which makes use of insight for sadomasochistic purposes. Another, occasionally related phenomenon, seen more with adults than children, is that of speaking with insight during the analytic session, but behaving outside analysis as if having no insight.

Different ego structures and functions associated with thinking, memory, self-observation, and judgment play a part in the formation of insight, which is an end result rather than a primary function of the ego. But ego functions that can contribute to insight are not themselves insight. This is illustrated by Freda A., who began treatment at six years five months. The indexing of her case was done at seven years ten months:

Freda asked the therapist how he knew she had loving feelings, then said that she sometimes called mommy and daddy "big, fat elephants and muck," adding, "One day I like them and one day I hate them." Freda commented that part of herself wanted to come to treatment to find out why she felt "bad: like half of me wants to come and the other doesn't; half of me wants to find out why I feel bad and the other half doesn't." In another session Freda related that she didn't like swimming but did like "running, jumping, cars," and then, looking startled, she said, "Funny, they are all boy things. Gee, there must be something wrong with me, these are all boy things."

Freda's comments seem primarily to demonstrate self-awareness and its use rather than insight. It is possible to have a highly developed capacity for self-observation as distinct from insight. This child has the capacity to observe what is going on inside her so that she can make pertinent self-observations about her ambivalence. Her observations do not lead her to know why her ambivalence is present, however, and we cannot say that she has insight.

ANNA FREUD   Freda has insight into the fact that there is something wrong with her; she has *Krankheitseinsicht*—but the term is meaningless without knowing to which elements her insight extends.

Joyce, an eight-year-old patient, would say to the therapist, when bringing in material, "I know what you are going to say," and then usually gave an appropriate interpretation. In regard to insight acquired in the analytic process, Joyce seems to be applying on her own behalf what previously had to be provided by the therapist— that is, an understanding or an interpretation which she is now making for herself. We can look on this as an identification with her therapist, though she is still saying it is her therapist's idea and not her own. Possibly this example shows an intermediate step in the development of insight. This example can also be understood differently; perhaps Joyce, though able to interpret her own motivation, still needed to defend against this knowledge by attributing it to her therapist's view of her. She may have been using one piece of insight to defend against another, to protect herself from a narcissistic injury.

A patient may merely take something over from the therapist and apply it to himself with a greater or lesser degree of conviction or meaningfulness. He may not have real insight but may, rather, attempt to placate the therapist by taking over his words, which are then made essentially meaningless.

The insufficiency of insight into motivation as a therapeutic agent is clear in disturbances that are ego-syntonic, which do not cause the child any discomfort. A child may have insight into his strong wishes and feelings and into his inability to postpone gratification or accept substitute gratification. Yet he may have no wish to change or may wish to change only the external world rather than himself. The problem is common in children.

There are also ego-dystonic experiences which are modified in treatment by the therapist's interventions and which are not directly related to insight as such. For example, the child may realize that a wish which was unconsciously felt to be threatening is not so dangerous after the analyst has shown that it can be talked about. This is not insight, although the child is relieved. The therapeutic agent in this situation is not primarily the acquisition of insight into motivation. Instead, it is the confronting of a more mature part of the ego with notions that were felt to be dangerous on an earlier developmental level. A distinction exists between the development of insight as a result of the analytic work and the use of insight as a part of the analytic process or as something that can foster further analytic work.

The development of insight as a consequence of analytic work depends on the presence of an ego-dystonic, ego-alien, uncomfortable experience. In child analysis this may involve making known to the patient elements which are painful and denied, such as the anxiety in a symptom or situation, feelings of guilt or shame, and other painful aspects of himself that are not accepted into consciousness or covered up at the outset. This acceptance must be worked at in the analysis, for the patient will frequently defend against it. The child may then gradually become aware of a conflict and its associated unpleasantness, which can result in an increase in his self-observation, self-awareness, and subsequently his insight.

9

Reaction to Interpretations

The effect of interpretation on patients differs for a variety of reasons. The interpretation may, for example, lessen or increase the resistance of the child. The particular reaction tells something about the child's personality, especially his defensive organization, which is of great importance for the conduct of the analysis.

The patient may react to interpretations in a particular way because of deficiencies in the therapist's technique. The interpretations may be badly phrased, wrongly timed, useless, or inappropriate for one reason or another. Reactions to interpretations may be connected with the patient's characteristic and habitual ways of responding, reflecting his personality in general and his defenses in particular. When offering an interpretation, the therapist should always take into account the organization of the particular patient's personality because it affects the patient's receptiveness to interpretations.

ANNA FREUD   The patient's response to interpretation takes many forms. For example, the patient may respond by providing more material after the interpretation has been given. In many cases this means an easing of the repressive forces, permitting more material to come to the surface. However, if too much material comes through, it may point to a vulnerability of the defensive organiza-

To Index: Describe characteristic or habitual ways in which the child reacts to interpretations (e.g. by providing more material, change in play, silence, manifesting anxiety or aggression, acceptance). Record the timing of the child's responses to interpretation, whether immediate or delayed, together with any other significant features of the child's reaction. Note changes during the course of analysis and exceptions to the child's habitual way of reacting.

tion. A change in the child's play may signal displacement and give evidence of the use of play as a defense by the child. A reaction such as silence points to the use of denial. Manifestations of anxiety or aggression may render the child vulnerable if the defenses are approached at all. The acceptance by the child of everything in the interpretation suggests a tendency to passive compliance. All these reactions to interpretations suggest that the analyst can make use of them in order to know more of the way in which the patient's personality and defensive structure are organized. They provide another way of going from the surface to the depths.

One type of response is shown by Katrina L.'s treatment, which began when she was six years one month old and was indexed one year later:

Throughout the first year of treatment Katrina frequently reacted negatively to interpretations. These reactions varied from shouting to silence the therapist and holding her ears with her hands, to aggressive outbursts directed against the therapist, such as spitting, hitting, kicking, or throwing objects at him. At other times Katrina's aggressive outbursts in response to interpretations were directed less at the therapist and consisted of throwing things onto the floor or across the room. On yet other occasions Katrina threatened not to come to treatment any more if the therapist continued to talk, that is, to interpret. These reactions were most noticeable in response to interpretations concerned with Katrina's defense of externalizing her feelings of worthlessness as well as her strong use of denial.

Katrina showed a kind of panic in response to interpretations. For this patient panic occurred particularly at the beginning of treatment, a characteristic response of many children whose attitude to treatment is determined by a feeling that they are being punished or attacked. Such children may react in this way for long periods in response to any attempt at interpretation. Many children react aggressively to acute guilt feelings as well as to acute anxiety. Often an aggressive response to guilt feelings represents a form of identification with the aggressor where the aggressor is the attacking and criticizing superego introject.

Although the reaction demonstrated by Katrina occurs most frequently in the early stages of analysis, it is possible to find such reactions later on, when the patient for one reason or another reverts to this mode of response. He falls back on the old defenses because he experiences massive anxiety or other painful affects stirred up by the interpretations when they touch on a particularly sensitive theme.

Another facet of a child's habitual reaction has to do with real limitations in his capacity to accept an interpretation. For example, a particular child may be able to accept an interpretation only if it is put as a story about another child or in the form of "How difficult it is for you to do this or that." Such devices enable the patient to maintain his self-esteem while accepting the interpretation. These aids to interpretation must often be used, because the therapist has to consider the ego's state of readiness to accept an interpretation as well as its tolerance for the content of the interpretation. The phrasing of interpretations, though extremely important, is not a sufficiently understood subject. Many questions have to be answered in this area, such as whether effective interpretations can be given by telling stories about another child or by reference to figures in a doll "family." Such interpretations are known to provide relief, but it is not known whether they lead to insight if they are not specifically connected with the person of the child himself.

Another response, the use of somatic symptoms, is illustrated by the case of Jerry N., who began treatment aged four years four months and was indexed two years later:

Jerry frequently accused the therapist of giving him a "tummy-ache" with her interpretations. He sat grasping his abdomen and refused to listen to what the therapist said. He also developed headaches, which he accused the therapist of causing. He used these as resistance against interpretations of sexual material.

ANNA FREUD   In this case the child defends himself by somatic means. I am sure that when Jerry is confronted with sexual material, he really experiences a tummy-ache or a headache, and these are his attempts to ward off unwanted thoughts and feelings. Naturally these somatic manifestations come into the analysis as resistances.

Sometimes an interpretation by the therapist is felt by the patient to be an attack of some sort. If so, the therapist may need to reformulate the interpretation. However, the patient's tendency to use denial or similar defenses may necessitate a certain insistence by the therapist on the interpretation, in order to get it through to the patient. Quite apart from the necessity for working through by means of the repetition of interpretations in different forms and different contexts, the therapist may have to repeat an interpretation in a different form simply to make it more acceptable to the patient.

10

Transference

The term *transference*, derived from adult analysis, refers to the way in which the patient's view of and relations with his childhood objects are expressed in his current perceptions, thoughts, fantasies, feelings, attitudes, and behavior in regard to the analyst. Especially in the analysis of children, transferences may reflect aspects of present-day relationships with important objects, in particular the parents.

Because of difficulties in defining transference, the term tends to be used in a broad sense, to include a number of different forms, as well as processes of externalization in which the therapist may represent different aspects of the child's personality, such as aspects of superego, of introjects, of instinctual strivings, of self-representation. In externalization, any aspect of the person is attributed to the external world. The term *projection* often has a more restricted meaning, referring to the attribution to another person of a wish or impulse of one's own toward that person, which is felt by the subject to be directed back against himself (he thinks or says, for example, "I do not hate him; he hates me"). Projection can be regarded as a specific instance of the wider class of externalization.

The term *transference*, used loosely, is often treated as a single phenomenon. However, four different types of transference can be distinguished here: transference predominantly of habitual ways of relating, of current relationships, of past experiences, and transference neurosis.

To Index: Record material relevant to transference in the widest sense of the term. Include externalizations when these play an important part in determining the relationship of the child to the therapist.

These are not rigid categories. Difficulties arise when theoretical concepts are approached as absolutes into which the therapist attempts to fit the observed clinical material. In a sense, the clinical observations are the absolutes in this context, and when the therapist comes to formulate his ideas, he does the best he can to make use of a set of theoretical categories which may be relatively imprecise, although adequate for clinical purposes. Although the categories overlap, it is valuable clinically to attempt to establish which category best fits a particular manifestation of transference, so as to attain some precision in a complex area.

Transference of habitual modes of relating

Modes of relating often seen in the earliest sessions of treatment may later become transference in a stricter sense. Examples are the tendency to make sadomasochistic relationships and the tendency to placate. A habitual mode of relating is exemplified by the attitude of the child who is frightened of policemen, doctors, or anyone in uniform or in authority and who begins treatment by being frightened of the therapist. Such fear might occur when a patient who habitually externalizes onto adults critical aspects of his superego relates to the therapist in the same way as to any other adult. This behavior would be a character transference.

The distinctive features of character transference are further exemplified by the adult patient who appears late for an analytic session. The lateness may be the consequence of a specific transference arising in treatment, perhaps from activation of anxiety about a homosexual attachment to the therapist. It may, however, simply reflect a characteristic tendency in the patient to be late. Psychodynamically, such fixed patterns are based on earlier relationships (or defenses against earlier object-directed impulses) and can be understood in this way in the course of analytic work. What is important

To Index: Show ways of relating to and attitudes toward the therapist which appear to be habitual and characteristic for the child. Seek aspects of the child's relationships to people (or to special groups of people) which are not specific to the therapist in any way but are aspects of character, insofar as one can speak of the child's personality having been formed.

in the analysis is that the residues of earlier relationships have spread to the world as a whole and attained a degree of autonomy. The therapist is confronted with the technical problem of how to facilitate the revival of the earlier relationships and catch them in their "live" form as opposed to their fixed form.

ANNA FREUD   This point can be seen in treating a child who forgets and loses everything. He forgets everything in the consulting room, which might have a definite transference meaning. Most analysts would say, "Of course, you wanted to stay with me and so you left your cap (or your penknife or pencil)." Then the analyst hears that the child leaves his cap and penknife and pencil everywhere—in school, on the bus, at home—and it can be seen that it simply isn't true that the child wants to stay in all these places. The whole thing has a completely different meaning and only comes into the analysis as a fixed symptom. The point is that when the analyst first sees that piece of behavior, there is no way of knowing at the time whether it is the one or the other. This particular patient demonstrated by losing inanimate possessions how "lost" he felt in regard to his parents. He lived with his father, who paid insufficient attention to him, and had actually "lost" the mother to whom the boy was deeply attached (except for rare visits).

Character transference involves relating in a habitual fashion to a whole category of persons. During the course of treatment the therapist hopes to be able to find a change in the quality of the relationship so that the specific person of the therapist becomes invested in a more focused way in the transference. There are technical problems in transforming character transferences into more emotionally loaded transference relationships. An example is the treatment of the child who habitually mistrusts everyone and commences analysis by mistrusting the analyst. The analyst might point out the child's mistrust and suggest that he may have good reason for being mistrustful because he has been disappointed by grown-ups in the past. It is an error to treat these habitual modes of relating as if they were full-fledged transference manifestations or even aspects of a transference neurosis, even though they are categorized as forms of transference in the broadest sense of the word.

Children have a continuing dependent relationship with the parents in the present. This complicates the task of distinguishing between a fixed pattern of behavior used with parents and adults in general and the specific revival of a past experience within the context of the treatment situation.

In the treatment of Michael B., indexed when he was seven years eight months old, after nearly two years of analysis, habitual modes of relating were transferred:

Michael's great problem when he commenced treatment was his fear of involving himself in relationships in case he should be abandoned. He defended against his anxiety by being as unpleasant as he could, thus inviting the object to reject him. The therapist felt that although the necessity to invite rejection had been diminished by treatment, Michael may still have had a tendency to retain this defense against close relationships.

Michael used habitual modes of relating as a defense against anxiety. When a habitual mode of relating appears in the patient's response to the therapist, an opportunity arises to show the patient the nature of his defense. The analyst may show the patient the contradiction within himself between the wish to be emotionally involved with the analyst and the fear of being involved, pointing out what the patient does to protect himself against involvement.

Another mode of relating is that of Esther L., whose case was indexed when she was nine years eleven months old, slightly more than a year after her analysis began:

One of the main features of Esther's object relationships was her need to defend herself against anticipated disappointments and rejections which she had previously experienced on both preoedipal and oedipal levels. Her parents had given a history of her past tendency to form friendships with children who would reject her. In treatment she showed a marked degree of self-sufficiency, and it became apparent that this, as well as her need to keep herself busy with a variety of activities, was her way of avoiding the rejection and the disappointment she expected should she ask for help or attention. As the analysis of this defensive attitude proceeded, Esther gradually became able to make demands on her therapist, and she recreated a situation in which she would provoke rejection or experience disappointment by making requests that could not be granted.

Esther's initial defensive posture is a good example of a habitual mode of defense used in relation to the therapist as well as to all her current objects. The defense was against disappointment and rejection, and with analysis of the defensive attitude, the underlying wishes were regressively revived in relation to the therapist, on whom they became focused. The difficulty in distinguishing between habitual modes and other revivals of the past is compounded when everything that happens between patient and therapist is called transference.

The inclusion of habitual modes of relating here is somewhat ambiguous. Sigmund Freud used transference to refer to the spontaneous development within the analysis of a libidinal relationship revived from the past. Later authors broadened the concept of transference by including various modes of relating, among them relatively autonomous habitual defensive attitudes as they appear in the analytic setting. Habitual modes of relating are not transferences in the earlier, stricter sense and can be considered transference only if the term is used in the widest possible way. An important clinical distinction between habitual character attitudes and the transference evolves in the course of the analysis. Although habitual modes of relating are not specific to the transference relationship, they may involve a great deal of intense affect and action directed toward the therapist.

Transference of current relationships

Current preoccupations transferred to the therapist may be largely reality-related, such as the child's regressive reaction to the birth of a sibling, or they may be a product or manifestation of the child's current age-appropriate level of functioning, such as the appearance of oedipal strivings as a consequence of the child's progressive development. The criteria for such a transference are that the preoccupations of the child relate to a real object or objects in the present and that their manifestations in the analysis represent an extension or displacement from that object. Such a relationship to the therapist has the predominant quality of a displacement or "extension" in the present rather than that of a "revival" from the past.

The distinction between the relation to the therapist as an exten-

---

To Index: Show the displacement of current wishes, conflicts, or reactions into the analytic situation or onto an involvement with the person of the therapist.

sion of the present and as a revival from the past cannot always be clearly maintained or easily made. The therapist attempts to gauge the distinction in terms of the predominant quality by the feel, flow, and development of the material. It cannot be assessed only by the feeling that something is very real in the here and now, because that feeling is typical of all transference reactions. The child who enters a new phase of psychosexual development obviously differs from the child who has regressed within the analytic relationship. Thus a child in the oedipal phase may bring oedipal feelings and conflicts into the analysis, where they should be seen as extensions of current involvements rather than as a revival of the past. The current oedipal relationship with the parents is displaced or extended into the analysis rather than being reactivated.

A distinction must be made between, on the one hand, the revival of something from the past within the analytic situation and as a consequence of the analytic process and, on the other, the extension into the analysis of something currently active in the patient's life. Current relationships extended into the analysis include regressive as well as phase-appropriate manifestations, a "spillover" into the analysis.

One form of transference of current relationships, which should be distinguished from the transference of past experiences, is consequent on the permission to express offered by the analytic situation. For example, a child of five, after some hesitation, allowed himself to shout at the therapist, obviously enjoying the experience, though somewhat frightened by it. After a while he remarked, "Mommy would never let me shout like that at home." This need be neither regression in the analysis nor transference. However, it can be a spillover of an impulse which the child felt to be prohibited at home; because the prohibition had not yet been fully internalized, the child could allow himself to express his wish to shout in the treatment room. When the therapist indicated that she could accept in an uncritical way the child's wish to shout, the child could respond to a different, externally provided ideal for himself, one which allowed him to feel safe and free from the threat of punishment in his relationship to the therapist. It may be a relief to a child to bring such material to the therapist, who is not such an important and highly invested object as is, perhaps, the mother. The permissiveness of the analytic situation allows more open expression, not because the therapist has really become the most important person in the child's life, but because she is a less important person.

The difficulties involved in regarding analytic material as transference of current relationships are illustrated by the example of Andy V., a boy who was two years six months old at the beginning of treatment and three years two months at the time of indexing (Bolland and Sandler, *The Hampstead Psychoanalytic Index*):

When his father started a new job which entailed his absence from home one night each week, Andy was markedly negative toward the therapist, particularly on Fridays, and often told the therapist to shut up, that he did not like him. This was seen as anger at the father's absence transferred to the therapist.

In this example, the child felt angry with the father for going away. The therapist felt that the child was angry with him before the weekend break because he transferred some of his feelings from a current situation with the father onto the therapist. A current situation impinged on the child, anger was aroused, and a similar situation in the analysis stimulated anger toward the therapist.

The example of Andy may not be transference of a current problem at all but may be a defense, by means of displacement, against the child's angry feelings toward his father. It would have been a displacement only if Andy had managed to lessen his anger with his father by doing what he did in treatment. What may appear at an early stage of the analysis as a manifestation of current problems may later be understood differently. For example, the anger with the deserting father might cover an earlier anger with the abandoning mother.

A further difficulty in distinguishing different forms of transference occurs when the child acts something out with the parents as a result of the analytic work. It may be unclear whether this is acting out as a consequence of the analysis, or whether the child is bringing some aspect of his current interaction with the parents into the analysis. The spillover phenomenon operates both ways.

A little girl was referred for analysis because of a profound reaction to the birth of a second child. During treatment, when a third baby was on the way, she became extremely angry about the new child "inside Mommy's tummy." The anger certainly referred to a current situation, but it also involved the whole of her disturbance in which the revival of the past was contained. What was predominant was a current problem which was carried over into the analysis. The patient hammered the male therapist's abdomen because she was very angry about the pending arrival of the new child. Her disturbance had begun with the arrival of the first sibling, however, and it would normally be expected that the past experience would be relived in some way in the analysis. Both a current and a past, revived reaction to the mother's pregnancy entered into the analytic material.

ANNA FREUD   What brings into the analysis material about the wish to destroy the baby? If the mother had not now been pregnant, would the material in the analysis at this time have turned to the anger about the previous pregnancy of the mother? Or is it the current event at home, the mother's present pregnancy, which brings the whole thing into the analysis? With children the material is quite often activated by a current event, so that it really comes into treatment like an intrusion. That is one of the reasons the whole procedure of child analysis often appears to be less orderly than that of adult analysis. It is not only determined from inside but also determined by outside events very much more than with adults.

This case illustrates the problems raised by the fact that regressive manifestations shown at home may themselves involve a revival of the past and may then be displaced onto the person of the therapist or onto the analytic situation. This situation differs from that in which something emerges spontaneously in analysis as a result of the analytic work, as happened in the case of Michael B.:

When Michael felt anxious about his parents' love, he would ask for oral satisfaction. For example, one month before his second sibling was due, he began to insist on having orange juice in the waiting room every day before his session.

ANNA FREUD   This is a spilling over of behavior, because surely at that time he had regressed and was more orally demanding at home and elsewhere, and the demands spilled over into the treatment. This spilling over is what is meant by the extension into the treatment situation. It is not a defense, in the sense that by demanding the orange juice at the clinic he succeeds in being less demanding at home.

Michael's example illustrates the therapist's need to determine whether the behavior in question occurs only under specific circumstances, such as at home or in the analytic situation, or whether it occurs everywhere and with everyone. If behavior is ubiquitous, it can be understood either as a habitual mode of relating or as a manifestation of regression.

The case of Ilse T. illustrates the complexity of childhood transference manifestations. She was four years eleven months at the start of treatment and was indexed when she was six years six months old:

On occasion Ilse's fear of her father was transferred onto the therapist, with the roles reversed. She would scold the therapist for her naughtiness, shout at her, or take the part of an exacting teacher (her father taught her Hebrew and English at home) and demand obedience. Ilse transferred to the therapist various aspects of her current oedipal relationship with her father, including her wish to be admired by him and her sexual wishes for him. For example, she wanted to exchange kisses with the therapist and sought excitement in physical approaches; she also wanted to make a baby with the therapist and was disappointed at not having her passionate desires reciprocated.

Ilse's case illustrates two separate modes of transferring a current relationship to the analysis. First, by scolding the therapist and taking the part of a demanding teacher, the child was transferring into the analysis her fear of the father while reversing the roles. What was extended into the analysis was something which had arisen at home. The way Ilse dealt with it in the analysis, by reversing roles, raises the question whether the reversal of roles was a defense against her feelings about the father-therapist. Or, because the child did not have the opportunity to reverse roles at home as she did in the analysis, she may have been trying out something in the analysis that she would have liked to do at home. Or again, such behavior may be understood as the child's chosen mode of expression, namely her only way of creating a situation in the analytic hour that could reflect the conflict inside her. In Ilse's second mode of transferring the current relationship with her father, namely through displacing developmentally appropriate oedipal wishes into the treatment situation, the child seems to have been more straightforward.

From the point of view of the treatment situation and technique, a parallel can be drawn between the prelatency child and the adolescent, because they share an intensity of developmentally appropriate reactions and conflicts, in contrast to the normal latency child. Current developmental turmoils may spill over into the analysis or be defensively deflected there. A special technical problem arises in the treatment of adolescents in that the therapist has to "fight for the past" because of the adolescent's enormous fear of regression. It is difficult for the therapist to evoke in the transference a revival of the past so that it can be analyzed fully, because as soon as regression threatens, negative feelings arise in the patient and enormous resistances appear.

Not only may the patient express feelings in the analytic situation about or toward the therapist which can be designated as the transference of current relationships and problems, but such spillovers may also occur elsewhere. Alternatively, it is something other than a simple spillover when the patient deflects attitudes, relationships, and problems into the analysis as a defense against experiencing them outside, feeling that the therapist is "safer," since at the moment direct expression (for example, to the parent) is in some way too threatening. In the course of treatment, the emergence of intense feelings about the analyst and of conflicts within the analytic situation is accompanied by a diminution of their expression outside treatment. What looks like a manifestation of transference neurosis in this respect is not so at all; nor is it transference in the narrower sense, that is, a specific revival of the past. In these cases it does not appear that the analytic process in itself plays a crucial role in the timing of the emergence of such material. The apparent transference represents a piece of defensive activity on the part of the child, a defense against the child's reaction to some external event or circumstance.

Transference of past experiences

Manifestations of the transference of past experiences may be considered to be derivatives of the repressed which emerge in regard to the therapist because of the analytic work. Such manifesta-

To Index: Refer to the way in which past experiences, wishes, fantasies, conflicts, and defenses are revived during the course of analysis, as a consequence of the analytic work, so as to relate to the person of the therapist in their manifest or latent (preconscious) content.

tions combine present reality, including the person of the therapist, with expressions of revived wishes, memories, or fantasies, such as preoedipal wishes for the exclusive possession of the therapist.

The case of Karen C., shows how this transference operates. She began analysis at twelve years six months; her treatment material was indexed when she was fifteen:

Karen turned the sessions into a repetition of her anal-sadistic relationship with her mother, through which it was possible to recognize her longing to reestablish intimacy. She bribed the therapist with gifts of food as mother had bribed her. She enacted being sick in the session, with the therapist tending to her, and imagined the therapist ill and being nursed by her. Karen tried to seduce the therapist to anal games, even to the extent of lying on the floor "as I did when Mommy gave me suppositories." Anal material was brought in, together with stories of illness and praise of mother, who never failed her when she was ill: "She would do anything for me, wipe my bottom or stay in the lavatory with me all night."

The example of Karen C. is ambiguous, because her behavior might equally well have been regarded as reflecting a general mode of relating to people at that particular time. It is crucial to determine whether the behavior arose as a consequence of the analytic work or not, but this cannot be determined from the description. The behavior could be regarded as a clear example of transference of past experiences if in the course of the analysis Karen experienced the revival of earlier anal wishes and if, despite having a fixation point at an anal level, she was no longer interacting with her mother in an anal-sadistic manner. If this were true, Karen's behavior with the therapist would not reflect her current relationship to the mother but could be regarded as a consequence of the analytic work and the analytic process. On that basis the example could be characterized as a transference of a past experience rather than a displacement from something in the present.

Anna Freud distinguishes between *fixation* at a particular level, at which level the child currently functions in regard to some aspect of his personality, and a *fixation point* at one or another level of development. Whereas fixations may change, a fixation point, once established, never disappears, although the child may develop past it. The fixation point represents a point in development to which the child tends to regress if conflict or pain become too great; it is also thought to exert a "backward pull" on the child.

ANNA FREUD It cannot be said that Karen, in the development of the transference, regressed to anal-sadistic behavior. She had lived on that level with the mother for a very long time and still did at the time of the analysis. She disturbed the mother at night, waking her up to demand food or to ask to be accompanied to the toilet, to have her bottom wiped, and so on. She disturbed any special occasion in the family by vomiting or by getting a sudden stomach upset. These were her symptoms. It was a question not merely of something which had become repressed and unconscious and which had then been revived in the transference. It was really that, with the development of the analytic work, the symptoms were drawn more into the transference. This process was greatly helped by the mother being enabled, through her own treatment, to stop this interaction, because the mother had kept the situation alive by playing her part in it. Karen's analyst did not play the same part, and so the whole thing became amenable to treatment.

One element complicating the distinction between the transference of past experiences and of present problems is the fact that the child develops a growing libidinal attachment to the therapist. Facilitated by this attachment, a current conflict at home might more readily spill over or extend to the therapist. Extension occurs because current conflicts usually involve past patterns of behavior which have been taken up or absorbed into subsequent developmental phases. This process is shown by the way in which a sado-masochistic relationship in the anal phase becomes structured and then persists, subsequently being absorbed into the structure of the oedipal phase and coloring it. It is not an arrest in development, because the child goes on to achieve phase dominance in the next phase. It is also not, strictly speaking, a fixation, nor is it a fixation point, because fixation points are silent and the concept of fixation points is intimately linked with that of regression. Absorption of past patterns into subsequent developmental phases is, rather, a persisting influence of an earlier phase on a later one. In the course of analytic work these earlier patterns find a more direct expression in terms of their repetition in the transference. It is not, however, absolutely clear whether such expressions are a revival of the past in the transference in the same sense as in the treatment of adults. A pregenital pattern may remain in the oedipal or postoedipal phases, finding more intense expression during the course of treatment rather than simply being released or regressed to in treatment.

Illustrating more clearly the revival of the past in the transference is the case of Esther L.:

During her resistant silences, Esther communicated her feelings of sadness, loneliness, and neglect by means of sniffing, finger sucking, facial expression, and general appearance. This behavior became particularly noticeable at a time when, following a holiday and a change of treatment room, she felt that she had been rejected by the therapist and replaced by another child. Her defensive self-sufficiency increased; she kept herself very busy with drawing and could scarcely speak at all. However, she revealed the feelings she was trying to deny in these nonverbal ways. When these feelings were linked to those she had following the birth of her younger sister, she responded slowly and gradually by seeking the therapist's attention in various nonverbal ways. She dropped things or could not find them unless the therapist helped her. She waited in the dark in the treatment room until the therapist turned on the light.

For Esther the interruption caused by a holiday and the disturbance brought about by a change of room led to a clear revival of feelings in the transference. These feelings were an aspect of the repetition of her past experiences around the birth of her younger sister. There were no discernible current extra-analytic factors which could have been responsible for the observed changes in the analytic material, but the changes in the analytic setting had a clear relation to the change in the child's material.

ANNA FREUD   What Esther was actually doing was not only seeking the therapist's help and attention but also changing her defense of self-sufficiency to an earlier state of helplessness. What the child repeated in the transference was a bit of her history. Prior to this development it was not clear what the self-sufficiency and overactivity meant. How did she acquire them? The therapist had no way of finding out until Esther repeated in the transference the experience of being neglected and deserted, defending against it by her overactivity and self-sufficiency.

Esther's behavior shows that when a defense is transferred to the analytic situation and is meaningfully interpreted within the transference, an earlier mode of reaction may become accessible to analysis. If the behavior is looked at from the viewpoint of transference of a defense, then it may illustrate a defense against the revival of feelings from the past, with a repetition, in this case, of the same defenses against the same feelings related to the same conflicts. This material could also be viewed as representing the use of a current defense against past feelings arising in the transference, so that it could be called a "defense against the transference," rather than a "transference of defense."

Also significant is the choice of defense for dealing with the repetition of past feeling states and experiences as they are reexperienced in the course of analysis. The child may use a relatively new defense, one which was not available to him in the original situation but which can now be employed to defend against the revival of the past experience. Adolescents frequently employ intellectualization as a defense against revived earlier conflicts such as concerns over violence and aggression; at an earlier developmental level intellectualization would not be an age-appropriate defense.

The choice of defense has important technical implications for treatment because it might not be appropriate for the therapist to link a defense with an early conflictual childhood experience if the defense is a later acquisition. Therapists often fall into a routine of interpreting a defense as being part of the reconstructed original experience.

ANNA FREUD The chronology of the defense organization is an interesting subject to study. One way to approach it would be to look at the analyses of adolescents who deal with their problems mainly by intellectualization, for example, by changing personal problems into a discussion of world problems. The analyst might ascertain what methods were used previously when the child had to deal with the same problem. It might then be possible to make a comparative study.

Transference neurosis

The concept of a transference neurosis stems from adult analysis. Whether a full transference neurosis occurs in child analysis is a matter of controversy which has research interest. The transference neurosis is a very special intensification of the transference involving an externalization of a major pathogenic internal conflict onto the therapist, so that the conflict is felt by the patient to be between himself and the therapist. His interest, attention, concern, and preoccupations center on the interaction with the therapist, and symptoms related to the conflict diminish in intensity or may even disappear.

In adult analysis a distinction can generally be made between transference neurosis and other transference manifestations. In child analysis there is usually significant transference involvement, but the evidence for transference neurosis is relatively sparse. The transference of past experiences may be regarded by some as transference neurosis, but the extension of the concept may weaken it.

ANNA FREUD   The difference between transference in children and in adults is that what the adult transfers and revives in the transference neurosis are object relationships of the past and relationships to a fantasy object, whereas the child, even in matters of the past, has the past relationship or fantasy firmly fixed to the persons of the parents. Therefore he has present-day objects, as opposed to past and fantasy objects, involved in his neurosis. [This has a number of technical implications. For example, the therapist would tend to interpret the transference from the mother of the present before referring to the past.] The question then is: How far does the child transfer past relationships and fantasies from the present-day objects to the analyst? That is the distinction. The child rarely transfers everything in the analysis because the objects at home are more convenient, since they are still important to the child. Therefore it is largely a matter of quantity, that is, of how much is transferred. If an adult patient was in a similar situation in treatment, almost all his problems would very soon be

To Index: Describe instances of the concentration of the child's conflicts, repressed infantile wishes, or fantasies on the person of the therapist, associated with the relative diminution of their manifestations elsewhere.

grouped around the analyst, around such issues as the holidays of the analyst and the analyst's other patients. What the adult patient had been enacting at home would be comparatively unimportant for the transference. It is a transference neurosis when, say, three-quarters of the patient's transference repetitions are focused within the analysis. The appearance of transference material in a young child's analysis does not diminish in any way the interplay with his current objects at home, or rather the living out of the neurosis at home, quantitatively speaking. The qualitative differences are the differences between real objects and fantasy objects in the child and the adult.

The transference neurosis, to whatever extent it can exist in child analysis, may be blurred by the degree to which the parents are still available to the child patient and needed by him as real objects. To borrow the concept of transference neurosis from adult analysis and impose it on child analysis, searching for analogues in children to the adult transference neurosis, may not be worthwhile. Instead, it may be useful to pinpoint the significant elements of the transference neurosis that apply and are appropriate. The process involved in transference neurosis in adults may occur for only very brief periods in child analysis. A process may last one or two days in child analysis which, were it to last for one or two months, might more readily be equated with an adult transference neurosis. It may be a waste of time to assess the child analytic case for elements significant for adult analysis, for they may have no exact counterpart in the child analytic situation; conversely there may be elements of significance in child analysis with no counterpart in adult analysis.

Similar questions arise about the occurrence of transference neurosis in adolescents. One possibility is that a full transference neurosis, in the adult sense, is not really possible for an adolescent because she is currently striving to break the ties with the parents and is acting out these relationships with others, externalizing her conflicts in the process. The adolescent's primary need is to distance herself from the parental objects. Toward the end of adolescence, a patient might go through transference developments which are more like the transference neurosis of adults.

Some therapists firmly believe that in children a transference neurosis can exist from the very beginning of treatment and that only transference and transference actions should be interpreted, claiming this as the correct approach to the technique of child analysis. But this view is an oversimplification.

ANNA FREUD   In the past it was understood that the appearance of a transference neurosis was a very gradual process which built itself up as a reaction to interpretations, to the analyst's "speaking to the patient's unconscious," and to the patient's growing positive attachment to the analyst. Thus the whole range of the patient's feelings was gradually brought into the new relationship, in all possible forms. Nowadays some analysts think that the moment the patient enters the treatment room he has a transference neurosis. This assumption does away with a great mass of detailed information about the patient.

A clinical example of what might be a transference neurosis comes from the treatment of Katrina L., aged six years one month at the beginning of her analysis, whose case was indexed a year later:

As treatment progressed, Katrina became more able to express her feelings and conflicts in the treatment situation. She showed herself a provocative, controlling child with many regressed behavior patterns and fantasies characteristic of much younger children. As her ability to express feelings evolved, her parents reported that she was more "perfect" both at home and at school. After about six months of treatment the parents said that her previous "hysterical" attacks had practically stopped and that she was at ease and seemed to enjoy life, had stopped being aggressive and provocative at home, stayed for all her meals at school, and was able to enjoy going to other children's parties.

Behavioral improvement seen early in the analysis of some children has often been called "transference improvement." There may also be a defensive "flight into health." In Katrina's case the improvement appeared only after about six months of treatment, following progress in the analytic work. The regressed behavior she previously had exhibited outside treatment became limited to the analytic sessions, and her behavior outside improved markedly.

Katrina's regressed behavior in the session can be understood either as the transference revival of something from the past or, alternatively, as the consequence of a "permitted regression" in the treatment situation. In the case of a transference revival, the relationship to the therapist undergoes a development, the material produced shows an evolution, there is a concentration of unconscious wishes and object investments on the person of the therapist, and something is revived from the past. The experience becomes all-absorbing and all-important for the patient. As a consequence, the importance of enacting or living out conflicts outside analysis is no longer so great; the therapist is, for the time being, the prime recipient of the early object relationship. In the case of permitted regression, a gradual development of a more tolerant situation in the analytic setting allows the child to feel less under pressure and less constrained. Feeling "Here I can regress," may allow the child to live out regressive wishes in the session and keep them in check outside. The child feels, "I can allow myself to behave in a less controlled and more childish fashion," having received "permission to express." This is an important point not sufficiently developed in the psychoanalytic literature.

ANNA FREUD   One of my early child patients, an obsessional, called her analytic hour her "rest time." All day long she had to make a great effort to keep her inner "devil" in check, but in the hour she could let him out.

Katrina's therapist saw the development in her transference material as indicative of transference neurosis, taking into account not only the intensity of the child's transferred feelings but also the changes that occurred outside the analysis. But the question remains of whether Katrina's transference to her therapist had the same quality of total involvement seen in an adult patient who, for example, falls head over heels in love with his therapist. It is conceivable that the "license" given in the analysis could account for all the phenomena and changes.

A permissive attitude in the child analytic situation contributes to the child's allowing his internal controls to relax. The relaxation may lead to behavior and material which is descriptively regressive, but which does not constitute a regression in the usual sense of the word. The child may be in situations at home and at school in which he is frightened to give in to infantile impulses or reactions, which he then consciously or unconsciously holds back. He works to maintain himself on a more mature level of functioning. Given permission and a feeling of security within the analysis, he may let his hair down. This is not, intrapsychically, a return to or a revival of infantile wishes, modes of functioning, and expression but, rather, a release of something currently present and "imprisoned" as a consequence of the child's fear of the reactions of external authority. There is a significant qualitative clinical difference between this behavior and regression proper. Some young children and many adolescents defend against the emergence of infantile tendencies, whatever the reason. Very often such patients, by using projection and externalization, perceive the therapist as a representation of an internal superego figure and resist any tendency to regress in either form.

Some therapists conceive of patients wanting to regress or actually regressing to a supposed ideal state of an all-embracing idyllic relationship between mother and child. This would be a Nirvana for the child or an ideal symbiotic state in which there are no unsatisfied demands, no painful feelings, and no frustrations. Such a state is a fiction. Even though in normal circumstances the very young infant probably experiences a state of well-being following on the gratification of his needs, the contentment is constantly disrupted by stimuli from within and without. Some therapists have built theories of treatment on the idea that nearly all pathology results from disruptions of the earliest state of well-being; they believe that the analyst can provide the gratifications that the patient is presumed to have missed early in life and that subsequently the patient's demands will diminish and the patient will retrace his development along healthier lines. This idea is reminiscent of Franz Alexander's theory of the "corrective emotional experience." It is thoroughly inappropriate as far as analysis proper is concerned.

Another example of transference neurosis comes from the case of Arthur H., aged twelve years four months at the beginning of treatment and fifteen years six months at the time of the second indexing:

Arthur's analysis pointed to a most intense relationship to the therapist, with many transference features, even in the face of real external conflicts in the home. For a long time he maintained an image of the therapist as an idealized parental figure. By the middle of the third year of his analysis there were many pointers to the development of what could be understood as a "transference neurosis." Arthur came to admit that if he allowed himself to experience pleasure, he might "lose" or "spoil" it. He initially rejected the transference interpretation that he felt the therapist could not tolerate his jealousy of Arthur's success or pleasure. However, Arthur subsequently revealed that often when he was enjoying something, such as football, he would have a sudden image of the therapist, feel awkwardly self-conscious, and his pleasure would stop. Arthur was told that the therapist would be leaving the country in six months' time. Working toward termination, Arthur verbalized his fear of hurting the therapist's feelings, which made clearer his equation of "giving up old objects" and "killing them off." Arthur then presented himself as "troubled" only in the treatment, whereas outside he achieved a great measure of self-confidence and assurance in his relationships. His feelings about treatment were understood by the therapist to be part of a transference neurosis because they were a revival in the analysis of old feelings of being abandoned.

The striking fact that it was Arthur's image of the therapist and not the image of the mother which spoiled all his pleasure speaks for the presence of a transference neurosis. It is possibly characteristic of the transference neurosis that the patient reports thinking and daydreaming about the therapist outside the analytic hour and the analytic setting.

Arthur missed a session in his analysis for the first time when he stayed at school to play football. Throughout the following weekend, Arthur felt miserable and anticipated the therapist's criticism for his absence. That Arthur was able to play football was owing to the progress of treatment; but his feelings of guilt and fears of retaliation were also related to the treatment situation. Arthur's expectation of punishment because of guilt may have been related to a conflict that was currently emerging in the transference; the anticipation of criticism appeared in the context of the analysis, and Arthur expected censure because he felt guilty about the pleasure he had experienced when he was away from the therapist. This reaction is different from the so-called negative therapeutic reaction, in which the patient punishes himself or fails because of an internal unconscious sense of guilt.

Because of Arthur's age (almost sixteen), it is doubtful if his material throws much light on the development of a transference neurosis in younger children. The capacity to develop a transference neurosis requires the ability to contain an internal conflict, a developmental task that is only gradually achieved. In younger children, the facility with which conflict is externalized interferes with the development of a transference neurosis because the therapist is also used for other purposes. In adolescents a further problem arises which is connected with the need to sever the ties with the parents; the adolescent fears regressive dependency in an intensive relationship with the therapist.

The child therapist is commonly confronted with a situation in which a patient's problem emerges in relation to the analysis, but it is unclear to the therapist whether the problem should be understood as a development in the transference based on the current analytic work or whether it is related to a change in the availability of the primary objects. The child therapist frequently sees an intensification of the child's feelings toward him when the mother is absent for a holiday. For example, consider the first eight weeks of treatment with a nine-year-old girl who began analysis with the anxiety that her mother would lose her, forgetting to pick her up after her session, even though the mother always did appear. The girl's anxieties were interpreted as indicating a feeling that her mother did not particularly care for her. After a few weeks the child said happily that she had found a way around her worry by coming to the clinic herself. In this way she saved herself the fear of waiting and the anxiety that her mother would forget her. Shortly after this session she arrived at the clinic too early. Pale with fear, she became extremely worried that her therapist had forgotten her completely. She had dealt with her problem in relation to her mother, but the anxiety appeared in the transference a few days later, centered on the therapist. It often happens that a child masters anxiety in one place, only for it to appear immediately thereafter in another place. Although the "other place" may be the relationship to the therapist, the anxiety does not always shift to the therapist.

During analysis the parents may be involved with many conflicts in many ways. Early conflicts may continue as live issues between the mother and the child. The conflict may have continued in its original form throughout the course of the child's development, or it may have been modified in one way or another. Thus a conflict over soiling may persist as such, or it may reappear in a new version, such as a struggle over cleaning teeth or washing. A new level of expression may be found, as when a conflict appears to be around phallic exhibitionism, but an associated sadomasochistic struggle with the parent is the real continuing issue. The availability of the primary objects to the child complicates the recognition of what is transference in yet another way. The child in analysis has the problem of dealing with his thoughts and feelings about his parents as they emerge in the analysis. Only gradually does the child develop the capacity to contain conflicts, fantasies, and impulses within the analytic setting. The younger he is, the more he has a natural tendency to action and to carry the products of the analytic work straight home. This tendency affects the interaction of the child with his parents and makes it difficult for the therapist to sort out reality, transferences, defense, and enactment.

It is important for the therapist to be guided in her interpretations by the current feelings of the child. Material should be considered, and if necessary interpreted, not only in relation to herself but, where appropriate, also in relation to the parents in the present as well as the parents in the past. In a sense the child analyst in her interpretations has to take up a variable position between herself, the present parents, and the internalized parents of the past.

The isolation of a conceptual entity of transference neurosis is a more difficult task in child analysis than in adult analysis. When a piece of analytic material from the past or the present becomes alive in relation to the person of the therapist, people other than the therapist may be involved; this occurs much more frequently in the analysis of children than in adult analysis. Moreover, the frequency of the child's pseudo-regressive responses to the implicit license to express offered by the analytic situation may complicate the problem of delineating a transference neurosis in child analytic work.

Changes in transference

Changes in the transference, if well observed and recorded, can give an overall picture of the important elements in the patient's developmental history as it has unfolded in the analysis. The case of Kevin C., aged thirteen at the beginning of treatment and indexed for the third time when he was eighteen years one month old, illustrates transference changes:

In the course of the third and fourth years of treatment, the main emotional involvement in Kevin's life was his girlfriend, with whom he repeated his

To Index: Summarize the stages through which the transference moves and develops during the analysis, noting, e.g., changes in the type of transference conflict and in the object that the therapist comes to represent for the patient.

early relationship with his mother. The analytic material was mainly concerned with the girlfriend, even when she lived in another town. The transference material seemed to be an extension of the involvement with the girl. The picture changed only at the end of the fourth year when the material centered directly on the relationship with the therapist, which became the place where the resistance was strongest. The oedipal conflict, both negative and positive, was transferred onto the therapist and worked through with her. The material now brought about home and school could be taken as a displacement away from the transference.

On occasion, the development of transference is reflected in the patient's involvement with a person in his contemporary life. Kevin brought such material in the third year of his analysis, in regard to the absence of his girlfriend. This material, quite clearly a repetition of an aspect of his early relationship with his mother, could be regarded as either transference to the girlfriend or a manifestation of the patient's resistance to the development of similar feelings toward the therapist. If regarded as resistance, his feelings toward the girl would be a displacement or extension of his unconscious feelings toward the therapist. The technical problem is how much to interpret the repetition of the past in terms of the relationship to the girlfriend, using the feelings and fantasies about the absent object as a path toward the reconstruction of the patient's unconscious processes and fantasies, and how much to take the material up directly as a resistance to the realization that such feelings are really felt toward the therapist. Therapists differ in their technical approaches in this respect. Adolescent patients bring a great deal of relevant material in the displaced form, and often they can stay in treatment only if this is tolerated by the therapist and not interpreted as a resistance to experiencing the transference in the present, as was true for Kevin. This procedure may, however, be technically appropriate only to treatment of adolescents because of the adolescent's fear of regression and his need to loosen his tie to his primary objects.

Transference was striking in the analysis of Tina K., aged sixteen years five months at the beginning of treatment and eighteen years nine months at the time of indexing:

Transferred feelings and attitudes played a most important part in Tina's analysis. The therapist's appearance reminded the girl of her mother's appearance, her continental origin, and her age. This stimulated passionate, mainly positive desires from the very beginning of the analysis. Tina expressed her homosexual wishes toward the therapist in letters, dreams, and fantasies. Her attachment was first understood and interpreted as a defense against her hostile wishes toward the therapist and also as a result of her fear of rejection, reminiscent of her mother's rejection of Tina in early childhood. An attempt by the patient to express more hostility gave way to intense feelings of depression. Her fear of losing the love object was excessive, but the libidinal aspect of Tina's feelings toward the therapist, her wish for physical contact, her curiosity about sexual activities, and her intense jealousy of the therapist emerged in the treatment and played a central part in it. Her need to see the therapist as a "perfect" person was interpreted in its defensive aspects and linked with her feelings that as a small child she had to see her mother as perfect in order to defend against disappointment. The homosexual transference was seen as defensive. However, during the second year of treatment, the transference became a predominantly clinging and dependent one, reminiscent of the relationship of a very young child to her mother. Tina's need to interrupt treatment at this point was partly the expression of her fear of reexperiencing loving, tender, and dependent feelings, originally disrupted by an abrupt separation from her mother. All of these feelings were reenacted and reexperienced in the transference.

In her analysis several roles were assigned by Tina to her therapist. They included elements of the real relationship, of the extension of current relationships, and of the repetition of past relationships.

ANNA FREUD   This case highlights the difficulties of apparent transference in the analysis of an adolescent. What Tina showed might well be an adolescent crush on the therapist, a sudden passionate involvement with a person who becomes idealized. For Tina, this was a real relationship. But was there really any possibility of showing Tina the repetition of the past in her current feelings? If so, would such an interpretation have diminished the intensity of her passionate feelings?

A distinction should be made between a "crush" phenomenon and a transference. Whereas the adolescent crush serves developmental needs, the transference in child analysis is usually, but not always, a revival of the past. In Tina's case, the crush can be seen side by side with transference manifestations. At times she also appears to be using the adolescent crush as a resistance.

Edward G. was three years one month old at the beginning of treatment and was four years eleven months at the time of indexing:

> Throughout treatment Edward transferred onto the therapist aspects of his relationship to his mother. There was no clear progression of the transference through definite phases but, rather, a tendency for certain transference features to occur in certain situations. When intercourse fantasies were predominant, the therapist was seen either as the castrating, phallic mother or as a positive oedipal mother, depending on how intense Edward's castration anxiety was. When Edward feared his mother's absence, the therapist was seen as the faithless, rejecting mother. She was also seen as the denigrating, rejecting mother when Edward's fears of his impulses to mess were uppermost, or when he felt unable to become the big, phallic man who could please and win the mother. Occasionally when Edward identified with the sadistic aspects of his father, the therapist was seen as the denigrated mother who was a "silly nitwit."

The material is typical of a three-year-old in that it depends on spillover from the relationship to the parents. Strictly speaking, the mother of the present is the transference object for the mother of the past, whereas the therapist may become a transference object by displacement from the mother.

The case of Lisa M., aged three years nine months at the beginning of treatment and indexed one year later, further exemplifies transference in a young child:

> Lisa transferred the oedipal features of her relationship to her mother (such as envy, jealousy, rivalry, and feminine identification) onto the therapist, while the preoedipal features of the anal phase (such as whining, clinging, and domineering) were much less marked. Sometimes characteristics of oral dependence were transferred, as in games of being the therapist's baby. Since the negative feelings belonging to the ambivalence of the anal phase continued to be enacted directly with the mother, the transference tended to be positive. Lisa's initial fear of the therapist and of being alone with her was seen as a transference of her fear of being seduced by the father, determined by her sadistic conception of intercourse. This fear disappeared after interpretation. She then for the most part transferred from her father her oedipal wish to be loved and admired, to please by being clever and competent, and to be given a penis and babies.

Lisa's material can be seen as a splitting of the ambivalent feeling toward the mother, which left the negative feelings directed toward the mother and the positive toward the therapist.

The cases of Edward and Lisa show that it is not difficult to describe what happens in transference. It is more difficult to identify and distinguish such factors as "splits" in ambivalence, elements of a real relationship, and repetitions of the past. With adolescents, in contrast to younger children, therapists face the additional problem of how to characterize those differences that are specific to adolescence, which change the way in which the transference is developed and handled by the adolescent. Transference in children under the age of five presents special features. It is important, however, not to ascribe too much to the child's age or stage of development, which may lead to neglect of other important factors.

The question of the resolution of transference, or the "myth" of the resolution of the transference, is relevant to transference development. Resolution of the transference implies that an active conflict involving the person of the therapist—one that represents the externalization of an internal conflict of some sort—should have receded as a consequence of the analytic work. The patient should also have a more realistic assessment of the therapist as a person, and the ties that remain to the therapist should ideally be less emotion-laden and conflictual.

In the case of a boy who had lost his father and was treated by a male therapist, two years after termination his mother reported that the therapist had played a large part in the boy's thoughts shortly after termination and that he had wanted to contact his therapist whenever he felt unhappy or upset. Subsequently, however, he made many relationships and got on well with his peers at school. Only when things went very badly or very well did he say that he would like to talk to his therapist, and then only to tell him about it. For the most part, the therapist seems to have been a benign figure for the boy, not a person who was heavily cathected, because the boy's emotional investments had moved to others in his daily life.

ANNA FREUD   This is an example of a resolving of the real relationship and not a resolving of the transference. In a case such as this, involving a fatherless boy, where somebody else takes over the father's role as well as the analyst's, the relationship is very mixed.

There are difficulties in keeping the two kinds of relationship—the transference and the "real" relationship—separate and apart. It is dangerous to neglect either of the two, and they really make sense only in relation to each other. The problem concerns neither the social relationship between patient and therapist nor the management of this relationship. Rather, it concerns the two sides of the relationship formed by the patient with the analyst—the "real" relationship between two people, on the one hand, and the distortion of that relationship through the transference, on the other. Although such mixtures exist in relationships outside analysis, in psychoanalysis the focus is much more on the transference aspects of the analytic relationship, and the analysis of those aspects is a major tool in the therapeutic work.

11

Other Uses of the Therapist

Besides transference, which enters into various aspects of the child's relationship to the therapist, other important elements in that relationship are made use of by the child. For some children nontransference relational factors are extremely important, particularly when the child has some sort of "ego defect."

Anna Freud takes the view that the other uses made of analyst and treatment situation should include the child's feelings and attitudes toward the analyst as a real person in the present and also the role assigned by the child to the analyst as an intermediary between the child and the parents. This particular role is one frequently demanded or hoped for by the child.

If the patient expects from the analysis that some change will be brought about in his external world but that nothing will be modified in him, his expectation may prove an impossible barrier to analytic work. According to Anna Freud the demand for this kind of role is often felt to be a hindrance in undertaking the analytic treatment of adults, or even children, who are in hospitals, orphanages, and other institutions. These are the patients who simply adhere to their implicit or explicit demand that the external world be changed. A positive result of the analysis is very often that changes in the external world are brought about by the patient himself. An example is presented by the child who asked for his bed to be moved out of the

To Index: Treat features of the child's relationship with the therapist not covered by previous headings. Include the child's feelings and attitudes toward the therapist as a real object, e.g. a person who gives the patient individual attention and understands him, with whom he can play, who is used as an "auxiliary ego," who serves as a model for identification, or who provides gratifications.

parents' bedroom. He was able to do so only after a relevant piece of analytic work.

Children who have severe emotional deprivations, of the sort often associated with grossly inadequate mothering or an absent mother, look to the therapist as a "real" object, wanting the therapist to fulfill their needs. Other children have an overriding wish for some specific external change, as exemplified by a girl who suffered from a deforming illness. Although she had many neurotic features, all she wanted from the therapist was a cure for her physical illness. Frequently in such cases the patient's interest in the analysis disappears once she realizes that her wish cannot be granted, but even if the analysis eventually gets going, the problem of focusing on the inner conflict is unusually difficult for such patients. In a less extreme form this difficulty is a common feature in the initial phase of the analyses of adolescents, who often prefer to see their problems as outside themselves.

A younger child was brought into treatment because she nagged her mother from morning to night that her parents, who had separated when she was two years old, should live together again. For the first part of the analysis it seemed as if the therapist's main function for the girl was simply to bring the parents together again. Behind this insistence was the girl's fear that she herself had separated the parents. When the fear was adequately interpreted, the problem was brought into the transference and could be analyzed.

ANNA FREUD   In a case of externalization, for example of conflict, what is taking place is not just a transfer of libidinal strivings. Something else is also occurring, and it is useful to separate the one from the other. Technically, it is enormously dangerous to interpret something only as a current object relationship when it is a manifestation of an internal conflict which is now externalized. The form of the externalization is naturally rooted in the patient's past relationships, but the externalization is not necessarily a revived object relationship emerging in the treatment. This can be illustrated by the simple case of an obsessional person who oscillates between the extremes of withholding money and generosity. He may transfer onto the analyst one of the two sides. To say then to the patient, "You see me as an extremely mean person," or to analyze the transference in terms of a criticism of the object as mean, is neither here nor there. The analyst has to analyze the situation as showing two attitudes in the patient, one of which has been externalized.

If the analyst is used as a new person, as a new love object, he can also be used as a new object of identification, as happens in children's lives all the time. This identification is not transference, although in every new relationship there are also transference elements because nothing is uninfluenced by the past. The therapist may serve as a model for identification, which may or may not involve elements of transference. There may be identification with the role of the therapist as a caring person, with some idealized image of the therapist, or with some real personal attribute.

The therapist should distinguish between early or transitory identifications and those that are more enduring. Identifications made in early life more often endure, but those entered into later in life need not be transitory. Identifications made in adolescence, with new ideals and heroes, sometimes remain. Although identification can be used for purposes of defense, it is a mistake to think of it simply as one of the mechanisms of defense. It is very much a normal developmental mechanism as well.

Another use made of the therapist concerns the nature of those changes in the superego and in the patient's ideals which allow the patient to feel better. Through his relationship with the patient, the therapist is involved in these changes. One possibility is that he is used for the externalization of an introject on which the patient depends for self-esteem or other narcissistic supplies. The more benign and tolerant qualities of the analyst may permit a modification of this introject, which is then reinternalized. Another possibility is that alternative ideals arise in the course of the analytic work, and the patient is no longer so dependent on his original ideals and on unaltered introjects, which persist but which no longer have their earlier power. Thus modifications may occur more within the ego than the superego.

Thus, the therapist may be used by the patient not only as a transference object but also as a real object, as a new object for identification, and as an object for externalizing inner conflicts or for the splitting of ambivalence. The therapist may at times also be used as an "auxiliary ego."

The term *auxiliary ego* is used frequently in describing the treatment of borderline or psychotic adults. The concept is also important in regard to the handling of blind children. In child analysis, the concept of an auxiliary ego may extend to the situation where the child is intellectually incapable of understanding something. When the patient asks the therapist to explain, the therapist may do so by providing information which the child's ego alone does not have or cannot grasp, simply by virtue of its immaturity. This is different from the situation with borderline or psychotic cases where there is a massive gap in ego functioning, which is filled by the therapist at the same time as other remedial processes are going on. Thus the concept refers to reality elements in the relationship as distinct from fantasy and transference elements.

ANNA FREUD   Analysts must regard transference as a distortion of the real relationship, or else the concept of transference will be lost. If, suddenly, irrelevant elements intrude upon a real relationship, the analyst should ask whether they come from the past or from unconscious fantasies. Of course, some of these elements may fit quite well into the real situation, so that they cannot be recognized for what they are. First, those that clearly do not "fit" or are not "appropriate" should be separated out. And here is a great difficulty in the analysis of children. In analytic work with adults many elements are obviously transferred—the analyst as an authority figure, as a parental figure, as a powerful person, to mention a few. With adults, such a transfer makes no obvious sense, because the analyst is not the parent. It does not fit, and it is clear that it comes from the past. But with the child many of these things do fit. The analyst really is an older person, he really is more powerful. So the analyst is in doubt about the source of these feelings and asks whether they truly are part of the real relationship or are part of a transferred relationship. But even with children, if it is transference, there will be some elements that do not fit. For instance, suddenly the therapist seems cruel, but in fact she has not been cruel; the cruel person is someone else. Or suddenly the therapist seems all-giving, but in reality she is rather depriving; the all-giving person comes from the past. This is the only way to sort out these phenomena.

In the situation of the patient who externalizes a conflict and brings it to the analysis in terms of a current object relationship, the therapist may interpret the externalization as a defense or may decide for some reason to interpret the content first. In making her decision she tries to assess what is uppermost in the child's mind and in his feelings. Fulfilling this criterion will affect her decision about how to proceed in her interpretation. If what seems dominant in the patient is his feeling of fear of the therapist's anger and his expectation of punishment by the therapist, the therapist may judge that the fear occurs because the patient has externalized aspects of his punitive superego onto the person of the therapist. The patient thus no longer has the inner perception of feeling guilty but, instead, experiences a fear of the object. This is quite different from the projection of his own angry wishes onto the therapist and calls for quite a different interpretation. The distinction between these two mechanisms is a crucial one, not always easily made.

The clinical example of Helen D., who began therapy at the age of eleven years eleven months, was indexed after a year and one-half of analysis:

Helen was from an orthodox Jewish family, and the therapist was non-Jewish. In the treatment, Helen often used this fact to express the fear that the therapist might not like her and might not understand her so well. Later this fact was also used in her conflict over freeing herself from some parental standards. Helen evolved a wish to remain religious but to be less strict about food laws. She also expressed a wish to become a therapist. This was understood as an identification stemming from her positive attachment to the therapist.

Sigmund Freud once pointed out that in transference patients can "cleverly take advantage of some real peculiarity in the physician's person or circumstances and attach themselves to that." This is true of children as well as of adults. Helen's identification with the therapist, who was of a different religion, could have been based on hostility toward her parents. It could also have been a defense against aggression toward the therapist. In the course of development children look for models different from the parents, however, and this is neither transference nor defense. Rather, it is a "trying out" of new objects and new models for identification, and the therapist is often used for this purpose. Yet another aspect of a patient's use of the therapist may be the wish to throw off cumbersome restrictions, such as the dietary laws followed by Helen's parents, and to identify with the more permissive aspects of the therapist.

Frank O. was aged seven years seven months at the beginning of treatment, and he was ten years one month at the time of indexing:

Frank's mother deserted the family when he was three years old, and his father took over the mothering in addition to his job. At the beginning of treatment a characteristic of Frank's relationships seemed to be that objects were used primarily for need satisfaction. Through the analytic work and the reliability of the therapist as a real person, Frank took a positive step forward in ego development, that is, in building and maintaining emotional trust in people irrespective of their physical absence or their nongratification of his needs.

In Frank's treatment the therapist was used at first as an object simply on the level of need satisfaction. A step forward in ego development was made later so that the child was able to consolidate object constancy and a higher level of relationship; the analyst was used as a real person, making up for lacks in the child. The question arises of the relation between the concept of corrective emotional experience and the occurrence and undoing of regression in the course of treatment. Was what had been observed with Frank one or the other?

ANNA FREUD   I think it was both, because what was analyzed was the great disappointment in the deserting mother. Frank regressed from the oedipal phase, reviving very primitive wishes to find a person who could fulfill his needs. That was the analytic part, but at the same time the analyst became a real substitute in his life for that missing mother, a person on whom he could rely, who would look after his most primitive needs, who would see that he did not get lost in the external world. It was the combination of this "corrective" experience of finding a better mother with the analysis of the relationship to the deserting mother which did the trick. Neither would have worked without the other. Such situations are frequent. They occur whenever the analyst takes into analysis a child whose father is missing. Many people would say that it is very good if such a child goes to a man for treatment. This is said, not because the man will be better able to analyze the child, but because the male analyst will be used at the same time to fill a gap in the child's life.

The use of the therapist to fill an emotional gap is particularly obvious with deprived children or with children who have lost some member of their family. This is also true when one of the parents is ill and the therapist is needed as a real person to substitute for the sanity that is missing at home. Crucial to treatment is whether a child is currently deprived in some respect or whether the deprivation occurred in the past. Current and past deprivations can lead to very different clinical pictures. Moreover, it is much less certain that a "corrective" experience can occur when the deprivation was in the past and is no longer current.

This view differs from Franz Alexander's. The question hinges on the nature of the child's structured adaptation to the experience of deprivation. The case of Dorothy J. shows something quite different from a corrective emotional experience. It illustrates, rather, the child's bringing of appropriate material to the therapist in terms of her current wishes based on a past deprivation. Dorothy was three years nine months when treatment began and five years five months at the time of indexing:

From an early age, Dorothy showed a great capacity to look after herself in response to her mother's inability to care for her during frequent and prolonged periods of depression. Dorothy's perception and use of the therapist as a real object was based on her wish that the therapist could be a substitute mother who would compensate for her own mother's inadequacies in caring for her. For example, she thought that the therapist should mend her clothing and lend her an umbrella. However, Dorothy seemed well able to distinguish the therapist as a real person. Whereas she expected her mother to be "forgetful," for example, and found it very difficult to "remind" her of her requests, she could perceive that the therapist was more reliable. She could also adapt differently to disappointments from the therapist, for example, by inquiring persistently after some requested play material if it was not provided the next day.

Dorothy used the therapist not only as a real person but also as a defense against her underlying impulses. Thus she shows how a patient may need to use the therapist in different ways. It is possible that children are more able to see the therapist as a real person than are adult patients. In a sense the adult patient, who lies on the couch and toward whom the therapist behaves differently, learns to allow more unreality to enter into his perception of the therapist.

ANNA FREUD   The reason Dorothy accepted comfort and care so easily from other objects, more easily than most children, was that she was used to them in the past. The role that she gave to the therapist might be the role her aunt had played in her early childhood when the mother was depressed. This child from very early in life accepted things from substitute objects which she could not get from her mother. Rather than transference of the libidinal relationship, there is in this case transference of a pattern. This is something different.

Dorothy identified with the benevolent and supportive aspect of adults in her environment, as shown by her capacity to look after herself from an early age. This maneuver is a reversal of roles. Identifying with a "benevolent therapist" is not transference but represents an attempt to find an adaptive solution to an internal problem.

Kenny K. was six years three months when treatment began and nine years three months old at the time of indexing:

There was no question about Kenny's transference reactions to the therapist. Yet the treatment relationship was indisputably a novel experience in that no adult, particularly a male, had ever taken his feelings and expressions seriously. In this respect Kenny experienced, perhaps for the first time, a relationship in which he felt understood by a man. In addition to this use of the therapist as an understanding object, Kenny seemed to use him as a valuing object. For example, in spite of his immense soiling problem and his idea that he was "no good," Kenny responded with pleasure to the therapist's remark that he was smart because he learned checkers so quickly. Kenny repeated this remark to his parents with pride. The fact that the therapist was a man was of use to Kenny during his long analysis by serving as an object for identification, a crucial factor for this boy in view of his father's unavailability as a masculine figure.

The child in analysis has a novel experience in that the therapist is an adult who takes his feelings and expressions seriously over a significant period of time. This has the result that the therapist raises the self-esteem of the child by saying, in effect, "I regard you as someone to be considered as important, and I am not going to dismiss you out of hand. I will listen to what you have to say." The therapist is available as a real person. Perhaps it would be more accurate to call this emotional experience "correcting" rather than "corrective." When the latter term is used, what is meant is that something in development which stopped as a consequence of a missing experience can be replaced by a "reliving" in analysis. For all children the therapist is someone very special. In certain children the experience of the relationship itself acts as a therapeutic measure, distinct from the understanding that comes from analysis proper. The experience of finding a new and stable object may help some kinds of deprived children to take the next steps in treatment and to benefit from the analytic work.

ANNA FREUD To be fully understood, a concept has to be looked at historically. In the past, there was a controversy between those who advocated offering an interpretation of the past and those who favored providing a corrective experience in the present. The proponents of the latter view specifically advocated that the analyst should leave the past aside and focus instead on the new experience. So it was that the concept of interpretation versus experience was born. Although the analysis itself and the relationship to the analyst contain a great deal of experience within which the transference takes place, that was not what was meant by the term *corrective emotional experience.* It was meant to indicate that it was technically wrong to place the emphasis on the uncovering of the past. It was said that in such cases treatment time was lost or regression to greater dependence took place, and analysts should therefore forget about the past and give the patient a new experience which would cure him. This view is unacceptable.

Among the other uses of the analyst is the child's assignment to the analyst of the role of provider. There are times when the analyst acts in this way, not only with children but with adults as well, as when adult patients complain about the cushion being too low and ask for another. That request may sometimes be analyzed as representing internal discomfort, but there are other patients to whom the therapist might simply give another cushion. The same applies to speaking: sometimes the patient is silent and the therapist decides to speak because he knows the silence is unbearable for the patient. Then a word becomes a gratification or a relief of some sort. The child therapist may need to take the initiative as a provider in order to keep the child in analysis.

Part Three

The Child's Modes of Expression

12

Bringing in Material

The child in analysis brings in his material in various ways. He may use verbal expression entirely, or he may play, paint, dramatize, or act out. In short, he uses different modes of expression. The form or mode in which the child expresses his material is significant for a full understanding of the analytic process. From the child's viewpoint it may not matter much whether he brings his material in the session, on coming or going, or outside the analytic setting by acting out in school or at home. From a technical standpoint, however, the mode of expression matters to the therapist because, among other things, the mode chosen reflects the degree to which the unconscious forces at work are accessible to the patient's consciousness.

The therapist aims in treatment to change those unconscious impulses of the patient that find direct expression in action into expression through thought or fantasy so that the child can exercise increasing insight and control. What is important in this context is not so much the content of the child's material as the form in which it appears.

The main modes of expression are verbal, nonverbal, or a combination of the two. They are technically and clinically important in child analysis. For example, special problems are presented by children in analysis who are difficult to handle and who bring in material predominantly in a nonverbal way. Such children give vent to a good deal of gross muscular discharge in their treatment hours and seem

To Index: State the main ways in which the child brings his material into the sessions either throughout treatment or at particular times. Note preferred modes of expression used to convey any sort of material or specific modes used to express specific types of material. Indicate whether material is primarily verbal, nonverbal, or both. Observe changes in the modes of expression the child uses.

unprepared to do anything else. Their inability to contain their feelings and impulses in words and in verbal symbols poses many difficulties in their treatment and raises the question whether they can be treated at all. The question of treatability is bound up with the question of the capacity of the child to bring his material in a way that is suitable for the analytic work and which allows communication between the therapist and the patient. The ideally treatable child might be expected to be able eventually to enter into a dialogue with the therapist. The child may bring material either verbally or in a nonverbal way that the therapist puts into words; either mode of expression may be suitable from the point of view of the analysis. What is necessary is that the child have the capacity to talk about what he has produced or think about it when the appropriate words are provided by the therapist. Implicit is the expectation that during the course of the analysis the child will move from nonverbal modes of expression to talking more to the therapist and to telling the therapist about his fantasies. This expectation may be derived from a model of adult analysis, however, and may not be entirely appropriate to the treatment of young children. In general, the therapist wants the child to move toward talking more, while at the same time she wants to see appropriate regressive moves during the analysis so that early material can find some form of expression, which may most appropriately be nonverbal.

Verbal material

Verbalization is the mode of expression which is ideally sought in the course of a child's analysis. Some children tend to produce verbal fantasy material throughout or in certain phases of treatment; others avoid this and restrict their verbal communication to descriptions of reality events. Such differences may reflect characteristics of the child's particular style of ego functioning, indicating, for exam-

To Index: Summarize briefly the dominant function of the child's verbal expression and, if it is known, the extent to which it is a general mode of expression or a manifestation of his resistance.

ple, his ways of thinking, his resistance, his defensive maneuvers, and so on.

A blind girl, Ingrid C., demonstrated in her analysis a variety of uses of speech. She began treatment at the age of six years four months; the indexing was done when she was eight years eleven months:

Ingrid's use of speech in sessions fluctuated. At times there was an outpouring of words, and it often seemed that this talk served to "fill up space." At other times there was a silent withdrawal usually accompanied by autoerotic activities. When during her second year of treatment Ingrid moved to elementary school, there was a change in the quality of some of the silences: no autoerotic activities appeared, and she was now able to comment on the silences herself with remarks like, "I don't seem to have much to say to you today."

In this child there was a great contrast between periods of much talk and periods of silence. It is common among blind children to use speech defensively against anxieties such as being left or separated; perhaps this was true of Ingrid when the therapist thought she was "filling up space." The fluctuations between outpourings and silences may be related to the means Ingrid employed to cope with anxieties. This is an example of the use of talking as a means of maintaining contact and perhaps also as a means of establishing the continued presence of the object; the content of the speech is irrelevant for these purposes. Later in treatment it appeared that Ingrid could better tolerate the anxieties around separation connected with silences. The evidence was that she no longer had to accompany her silences with autoerotic activities. Subsequently, silence seemed not to be an inevitable threat of separation and Ingrid could comment on the silence, showing her newly developed capacity for self-observation. The use of words as a reflection of the self-observing function in action, as a means of relating to the object, and as playthings, or their use in the service of resistance, all contrast with the use of words to tell a fantasy or a dream. What is shown here for a blind child also has application to sighted children.

The case of Victor C. raises points about an adolescent's use of speech. The patient began treatment at the age of twelve years six months, and the indexing was done one year later:

Victor communicated mainly verbally, and this seemed to be so pleasurable to him that he often found it difficult to leave at the end of the session. By the second and third years of treatment, Victor used verbal means exclusively and brought up his conflicts by reports on external events. For example, his oedipal problems and rivalry with his father were expressed in thoughts about the death of the pope.

The fact that Victor found it difficult to leave at the end of a session was linked by the therapist with the gratification the child obtained from contact in the session, a gratification perhaps related to the sexualization of some aspects of transference. In other cases such a reluctance to leave can have many different meanings.

Considering Victor's age, the changes in use of speech may be appropriately related to his progressive development. In younger children, the possibility of a skewed development of an ego function like verbalization must be kept in mind; such skewing is often observed in the analysis of obsessional children.

Frank O. brought up material predominantly through verbal modes of expression. He was seven years seven months when the treatment began, and his case, indexed when he was eleven years six months old, shows the different uses he made of his verbal ability:

Frank had an ability to use words in a very flexible manner: as sounds in a piece of symbolic play, as verbal symbols or imagery, and in a directly secondary process way. This verbal flexibility developed only gradually during the treatment. Throughout the analysis Frank brought an abundance of fantasy material, but almost entirely in the mode of actions and symbolic play. Near the end of treatment he enacted a fantasy with the curtains, accompanying this by an infantile voice. After the fantasy was interpreted, Frank brought material verbally for the rest of the session.

For Frank, verbalization in the treatment process had the function of putting into words material which existed previously only on the level of symbolic play, which he worked through in great detail. Once the enactment representing an unconscious fantasy was put into words by the therapist, the child was capable of working it through on the verbal level. The context in which this enactment or symbolic play appeared strongly suggested that it was the manifestation of a fantasy about birth. Perhaps such an enactment could be a highly sophisticated way of depicting fantasies about a child in the womb, rather than being a primitive communication which dates back to an experience of being in the womb.

Some therapists have the misconception that material which comes verbally is more true, or shows that the analysis is on firmer ground, than material that is brought nonverbally. Particularly in child analysis there may be times when nonverbal material, such as a play enactment, reveals an unconscious fantasy more directly than a verbal communication could. So-called confirmatory verbal material may actually be a compliant echoing of the therapist's intervention, something that is found in adult analysis as well. Another difficulty in child analysis is the gap in the ways of communicating between child and therapist, which results from their not being at the same level of ego development.

Silent or internal speech can find indirect expression in drawing, in dramatization, or in play. Play for the young child is an in-between stage, falling between enacting without control and putting into words as a precondition for controlling thoughts. A developmental task for all children is the use of words for this purpose. The child uses drawing in the same way as he uses play or dramatization: as a "derivative" which conveys content that can be interpreted. The analyst aims to assist the child to verbalize his feelings and the links between his feelings and his other experiences, thus making them more accessible to his understanding and control. Verbalization often enables the child to give the stamp of unreality to a fantasy, to understand that the wishes of the fantasy are only wishes in thought and not equivalent to action. The child can then better tolerate otherwise dangerous fantasies, adding to his understanding and control.

ANNA FREUD   What are the tools of the ego? What are the tools in child analysis for undoing structure as well as for building structure and secondary process functioning? We analysts may ask how other therapists work who do not, like analysts, direct themselves intentionally to the ego. For example, consider the type of treatment in which abreaction plays a large part. In a way, abreaction is also indirectly aimed at the ego, because through lessening the pent-up affect by abreaction, the ego has a better chance to deal with the remainder. Or we may ask how the interpretation of symbolic expression functions in a treatment based on this approach. The same question applies to the child who draws or models in treatment. Verbalization should be examined in the general context of ego tools and ego means, keeping in mind that thought and words are means of civilizing the individual, and that "putting into words" can be a substitute for action. I am reminded of a consultation with a mother who was very disturbed about her two-and-one-half-year-old boy. He had recently had some kind of a personality change, and she was afraid that this was because of her own actions. She could not stand it when he was aggressive toward his infant sibling, and she would become aggressive toward him. This made him more aggressive toward the baby, but frightened him so that he could not sleep. She did not know what to do with his aggression. His aggression toward the baby had two sources: first the angry jealousy of the baby and then the anger deflected from the mother. He did not dare to express anger to the mother, and so he hit the baby. He was also late in talking and could say only a few words. I suggested to the mother that she lend him a few very simple words and concepts and, with them, aim to bring about a series of changes. The first step would be to express to him, "It isn't naughty baby at that moment, it is really naughty Mommy." This would undo the displacement from mother to baby with the help of words. When she had drawn his anger to her, or made it clear to him that the anger was toward her, she could then say that he would want to hit her instead of the baby. He would then want to hit the person at whom he was really angry. But the next step—and she should have known after all that he would not do much to her—would be to teach him to say, "Naughty Mommy, cross with Mommy," which would be the step from action to complaining in words. Once she had brought him to that point, she really would have him on the way to dealing with his anger toward her. This child was only two-and-one-half, but this is the way the primitive ego gets hold of its impulses and gradually masters them. My father once remarked on the philosopher who said that the man who first hurled a word of abuse at his enemy instead of a weapon was the founder of civilization. That is really what analysts are aiming to do in getting patients to verbalize.

In very young children, and in children with certain kinds of pathology, such as nonspeakers, a verbal interpretation often does not convey enough to the child and may become meaningful only after being linked with a concrete representation, such as a play enactment of the mother leaving and the child crying. In such situations, a friendly tone of voice may mean much more initially than the verbal content of the therapist's intervention. Verbalization is not the only route to helping the child to reach an understanding of his problems and bringing him into contact with his feelings about them. There are pitfalls, however, involved in the nonverbal aspects of treatment, pitfalls associated with the degree of pleasure and gratification the child has in acting rather than in verbalizing.

Nonverbal material

Some children bring general or specific material mainly through nonverbal behavior and activities ranging from gross bodily expression of impulses and affects to much more "removed" or "displaced" activities such as play. Play itself covers many levels of symbolization and displacement. Play material may be used merely as a substance for hammering, scribbling, or throwing, or it may be utilized for imaginative and symbolic expression. In the very young child action and play are natural modes of expression; even in older children verbal communications are not without distortions. The inability of a very young child to verbalize has not quite the same significance as such an inability at the age of seven or eight. Often nonverbalization in a child who has the capacity to verbalize represents a defensive posture. For many therapists the verbal mode of expression is the most comfortable; they find it more convincing and technically easier to handle. Some therapists dislike a lot of motor activity. Some prefer to have a game to encourage another form of expression which is at a distance from themselves, so that they are not drawn into too close an interaction with the child. Because they prefer the game in order to defend themselves, their preference may interfere with the analytic work.

It is common for a very young child to express unconscious fantasies partly in play with dolls and partly in role play. When the therapist comments on the play, the child may become extremely angry and aggressive and leave the room. Such children can be pre-

To Index: State the extent to which the child brought material through actions and activities and describe the dominant features of the material.

cocious in their verbal ability, which indicates that it is not that they are unable to verbalize, but that they refuse to do so.

ANNA FREUD   The refusal of such children to verbalize or to permit verbalizing by the analyst may be defensive, because it is obviously the defense that creates the resistances. What is striking is that the defense does not go against action, even though the action can hardly be called symbolic and is a fairly direct expression of the underlying wish. It is so near to the original wish that the full defense goes against its verbalization.

Some children can allow themselves to enact something without paying full attention to it; the experience is permitted to come through but escapes the child's full awareness. Awareness may be linked with embarrassment or guilt; any verbalization which draws attention to the enactment may heighten such guilt or embarrassment and therefore stimulate defensive behavior, including defensively aggressive behavior. Although this phenomenon can also be seen, to some extent, in the adult psychoanalytic situation, for adults the role of verbalization is much greater and there is less scope for enactments that bypass awareness.

The self-observing function is related to the use of speech and the analytic process. A small child in treatment who refused to verbalize became angry at times when an interpretation was aimed at making her look at what she was doing. In fact, she resisted looking at the angry or "bad" part of herself. This does not mean that her self-observing function was not developed, but that it could not be mobilized in the service of the treatment, because of feelings of shame or guilt. Verbalizing for the child *can* have the effect of focusing the child's attention on himself, thereby stimulating the self-observing function and helping him to use it in the analytic process. Verbalization also can help the child to grasp something of the "technique" of being analyzed.

Play in child analysis is believed by many therapists to be the equivalent of free association in adults.

ANNA FREUD   If a situation is set up for a child in which free action is equated with free association, then the analyst becomes very busy defending herself. What the analyst should really pay attention to are the ways in which the child can bring material not dependent on the concept of free action. Not all the varieties of play in the analytic session come under the heading of free association. The choice of a particular activity may come under this heading, but playing board games or building model ships or planes are logical sequences dominated by the rules and needs of those particular activities. Building a model need not be defensive, but it is not comparable to free association, because it follows a logical sequence of activities. Fantasy play can reveal a great deal of material, but any kind of play can be used defensively. A serious obstacle in child analysis lies in the child's relative inability to remove the logical controls he has to exercise over thought processes without at the same time removing the similar controls over action. The adult can usually do this relatively easily.

Technical problems arise when a game or play in the session seems to be used purely for purposes of resistance and when repeated interpretation is not enough. A therapist may say to the patient at some point, "I am not going to play," if the child wants, for example, to play chess as a defensive intellectual game and the therapist knows that nothing else will then happen in the session. It is up to the therapist to encourage the child to bring up his material in whatever way possible. It is also up to the therapist constantly to assess the potential usefulness to the analysis of a particular activity. Thus, playing games for a period does not necessarily serve only resistance in the child. There may be some material which can emerge only in this way, or the child may need time to feel sufficiently safe and comfortable in the analytic situation before going on. In this regard an interesting question may be asked: Is it normal for the child to want to communicate during the session? Or is it a convention which therapists expect the child to accept from early in the analysis? Therapists make the assumption that if the child is uncommunicative, he is in resistance, but what they really mean is that he is refusing to accept a demand which they, as therapists, make on him, and with which they normally expect him to comply.

The fact that playing formal games need not always reflect resistance is illustrated by the patient who, after insisting on playing chess with the therapist, could only then show what had happened when he won his first chess game against his father; the father had thrown the entire set to the floor and angrily said that the boy's winning was a fluke. On the question of whether this material would have found expression in some other way if the therapist had been unable to play chess or had refused to be drawn into this particular activity with the child, the material probably would eventually have emerged even without the game, contrary to the widespread misconception that thwarting any activity in the analytic hour stops the child patient from communicating. Indeed, it is unlikely that the child always has a wish to communicate. Of course, unconscious wishes push toward expression in some derivative form, which certain analysts always understand as reflecting a wish to communicate, but there are many defensive maneuvers which might be conceptualized equally well as the expression of a wish not to communicate, not to be understood. Analytic work ideally leads the child patient to a wish for help with his problems, perhaps through understanding, and analysis of the defenses ideally brings about a wish to communicate. The same applies to adult analytic work.

The use to which a child puts the toys in treatment, whether for purposes of expression, communication, or defense, may be affected by the particular toys made available in the sessions. There are technical analytic principles for choosing which play material to provide for the child. Some analysts believe that the play material should above all allow for the maximum freedom of expression by the child.

ANNA FREUD   The emphasis on toys neglects one very important consideration. Child analysts all know that certain toys serve the production of fantasy better than others. But this ignores the division between those children who are able to produce their material displaced onto toys and those children who are not and who can use only their actual circumstances—either their own body or their analyst's body or real things—to act out their hidden impulses. Analysts know that it can be a progressive move if the child dismembers a doll instead of being aggressive toward the analyst. Providing sand and water, however, is also often a seduction to regression, and there is usually enough regression to be dealt with anyway. Historically in child analysis the initial idea was to choose toys for the child to make a so-called little world, in which almost everything in the real world was present in miniature form. No variation was allowed in the toys that were chosen and with which the child began treatment. These toys were part of the treatment setting, and they could be used by the child to express his fantasies. Quite apart from their use in this way, toys are used in quite different ways. They may express ideas of value, feelings of exclusiveness, or rivalry with others. They may, for instance, serve as missiles. The role of the toy as an instrument for analysis is greatly overrated. Whatever is provided is really only an adjunct to the treatment situation, and what is really important is what the patient and analyst say and how they relate to each other, what the child reveals, and so on. There is a point regarding play as an analytic tool which has always led to confusion. It concerns the difference between learning about the child by observing his behavior and then translating that behavior into its unconscious roots, and gathering analytic material which is produced relatively easily because it is disguised in free associations, in dreams, in fantasy, and in fantasy play. This difference has to be kept in mind with respect to play. Although it is perfectly true that one learns much by playing chess or by watching other activities, these cannot be equated with free association. I can also learn a great deal by watching a child at mealtimes or when he is undergoing a psychological test. The analyst as behaviorist can use pieces of behavior to extract unconscious meaning from them, for example to infer how the child deals with anxiety or with frustration. But this is quite different from free association or from the expression of a fantasy which results from an upsurge from the depths of the mind toward the surface because different conditions have been created which facilitate the emergence of the unconscious material.

The idea of making all kinds of toys available to all of the children contrasts with the practice at the Hampstead Clinic. There, specific toys are provided for the individual child in the child's own locker, in order to provide the most suitable way for the child to display what he cannot express in words. Toys are not so suitable when they are freely available on the shelves around the playroom, though some therapists maintain that the child's fantasies are demonstrated by whatever toy he chooses or picks up and that the significance lies in his action. The child may go on to other toys or activities which are not analytically appropriate but are used only because they have an intrinsic atttraction or a value for resistance. Thus the free availability of many toys lessens the effectiveness and the productivity of the analytic work.

Nonverbal modes of expression were used by Richard B., who began treatment at seven years eleven months and who was nine years old when the material was indexed:

During the first six months of Richard's treatment he went to the lavatory two or three times per session because of violent stomach aches. Later on, Richard replaced his visits to the lavatory with open anal masturbation during the session in front of the therapist. His lavatory trips came to be understood as his wish to tell about his "damaged bottom" which could not hold in the excrement.

Richard may not actually have had a wish to tell the therapist about his "damaged bottom," for his "push toward expression" may not have been conscious. In the case of children who run out of the room to act on an urge to masturbate or to urinate, the leaving of the room is better viewed as a bodily accompaniment of their feeling state. In Richard's case, a premature symbolic interpretation of his activity on the anal level might have been wrong, because what might actually have been going on was a conflict related to the phallic phase, a preoccupation with castration, which was put in terms of a damaged bottom.

Although a great deal of meaning attaches to Richard's repeated visits to the lavatory, to view these visits solely as Richard's response to anal excitation would be incorrect. They should be viewed, rather, in the context of an enactment of a fantasy with the therapist. It is true that such an activity is not always object-related, but in this instance it was. It was a symptom the patient brought into the analysis by involving the therapist, just as he had involved his mother at home.

Paul Q., who had begun treatment at three years four months old and was four and one-half when indexed, expressed unconscious content in play:

Throughout his treatment Paul made use of the faucet and flowing water to illustrate his fantasies and fears about his penis and its activities. When his castration anxiety arising from his concern about masturbation was dominant, he would clutch at the faucet, asking if it would break. He would anxiously start the water, still holding on to the faucet. At times when he was terrified by holes, he used the flowing water to help him temporarily to master the anxiety by stopping up the overflow hole in the washbasin, thereby flooding it. At other times, he gently turned on the faucet and told the therapist he was thirsty and that he thought she must be a teeny bit thirsty and want to have a drink with him. In this way he expressed what were thought to be impregnation fantasies.

ANNA FREUD   Materials like water and sand lend themselves to symbolic play. It is up to the therapist how to understand the symbolism and how to use it for interpretation. No one really has confirmation of how far a symbolic interpretation matches a fantasy in the mind of the patient, or how far it represents a fantasy in the mind of the person who interprets. Because symbolic interpretation is so open to the influence of the analyst's speculations, I do not like it.

Symbolic expression occurs in behavior and other nonverbal ways and is equally well manifested verbally, as in dreams and spoken fantasies. Of necessity, child therapists must be interested in issues related to nonverbal expression and must seek to learn how to bring about a shift from expression in direct action to expression in thought and words. With such a shift, even if the child continues to act rather than speak, he may become aware of an intervening thought that can be verbalized. The ability to verbalize may give him the opportunity to exercise some control over his actions and to understand his motivations better.

Tommy E. exhibited a defense against a wish, a defense he expressed nonverbally. Nine years seven months old when treatment began, Tommy was thirteen years nine months old when the material was indexed:

During a period in treatment when Tommy became increasingly aware of positive oedipal wishes in the transference, he came to his sessions wearing two pullovers, a blazer, and an overcoat. On one occasion he put on his gloves as well. This behavior was understood and interpreted as reflecting his need to defend against his wished-for sexual bodily contact with the therapist. He protected himself by an "armor" of clothing.

There are children who defend against their anxieties about being attacked by the therapist by putting on extra layers of clothing. In Tommy's case there was probably first a projection of a sexual wish toward the therapist, after which the child could then protect himself from his own sexual wishes by protecting himself from what he feared were the therapist's intentions. Other interpretations are possible, although the defensive aspect of Tommy's behavior is obviously the dominant one. It could be that Tommy was defending against not his projected sexual wish but rather his direct sexual impulses, which he had to control, possibly with a need to hide an erection as well. This boy was nearly fourteen and normally talked relatively freely, but in this period he could only be understood by means of his nonverbal activities. The adolescent process itself may have played a part in determining the choice of this mode of expression, one directly involving the body.

Mary G. brought analytic material into the sessions in nonverbal ways. Eight years nine months old at the beginning of treatment, she was twelve years old at the time of indexing:

Mary's appearance is an important way in which she brings material. It can almost be used as a barometer to indicate her mood. In addition, when she is looking to the therapist for specific advice and judgment about her appearance, she may wear a particular dress for the purpose. This is especially true in the case of the clothes chosen by her mother, which seem to Mary in one or another way to be unsuitable. For example, Mary came to the session preceding a Christmas party at school wearing a Dutch costume in which she clearly felt self-conscious and uncomfortable. She needed to show it to the therapist because she felt uncertain about showing any criticism of her mother's choice. Many important elements emerged from this incident, such as her fear and courting of criticism. Much later her wearing this dress reflected a hostile aim, a means of demonstrating that her mother and, in the transference, the therapist always gave her the wrong things. Throughout the analysis, transference feelings relating to separation and fears of criticism as well as material around self-denigration linked with guilt over aggressive wishes were expressed by the way she dressed and wore her hair.

ANNA FREUD   Mary could make herself appear attractive or unattractive, well-cared for or bedraggled, according to the feeling that struggled for expression in her. This was a nonverbal expression of how she was feeling about herself. Analysts see such expression often in adult analytic patients, as when changes in their relationship to the analyst are expressed not verbally but by the way they come dressed.

From a technical point of view, if material such as Mary brought in her manner and dress is expressed only in the patient's attire or appearance, the therapist may be reluctant to comment on this before the patient does, especially at the beginning of therapy. It may also be very difficult to understand the meaning of material which is brought without any verbal accompaniment. In young children, appearance and dress may be an indication of the mother's neglect of the child. But they may also be the child's way of accusing the mother. Because the child cannot do so verbally, she uses nonverbal defensive ways of expressing negative feelings.

A combination of material

The most frequent mode of expression found in child analysis is a mixture of verbalization and some form of nonverbal activity, as in play with puppets, in role play, or in any activity in which the child engages and in which he expresses content by both words and action. The different modes of expression employed simultaneously do not necessarily have the same function nor express the same content. Therapists often use the term *nonverbal* as if it refers to something specific, whereas in fact it covers a host of different kinds of expression, including drawing, dramatization, direct discharge through motor activity, the conveying of meaning by silences, and so on. Much can be conveyed by the tone of voice, which is not verbal but vocal. Even when referring to a "verbal" mode, the therapist should distinguish between something which is vocalized and something which may be written in the form of notes, stories, or essays. It is typical of certain latency cases that the child is able to express in written words what he cannot convey in the spoken word. Even the optimal mode of expression may have to be taken into account by the therapist in her own activities. Thus she may take part in play with the child and accept the role in which the child has cast her, not

To Index: Record child's use of a combination of verbalization and some form of activity as a mode of expression. Record any other modes used by the child, whether they are used throughout treatment or in certain phases only. Comment on function of the various activities, whether they function as a vehicle of unconscious content, as affective discharge, as a form of defense, or as an accompaniment to some other form of expression. Include instances in which the child brings in material predominantly through one mode (e.g. nonverbal means) and supplements it in a significant way by means of another mode (e.g. verbalization).

so much as a collaborator but rather in an effort to contact the child and to engage with him in the analytic work. The therapist may also give interpretations within the role she has assumed.

Candy, aged six, wanted to play "mothers and babies" with her therapist, giving the therapist directions and seeking a sort of physical contact, but not wanting the therapist to talk. Often with such patients, if one does not play along with the child, the material is blocked altogether and the child withdraws. Whereas with other children this kind of play usually leads to something else eventually, it seemed that Candy wanted only the gratification of contact. In the early phases of analysis, not only may playing as the patient wishes serve to gratify her, but the patient may need this activity simply in order to feel safe and sufficiently valued at that time.

A combination of modes of expression was employed by Helen D., who began treatment at eleven years eleven months and was thirteen years four months old when indexing was done:

> During her first year of treatment, Helen had a general pattern of behavior which was understood as a form of asking for help. She would begin the session by describing some anxiety or upset feeling during the day—for example, she felt one of her girlfriends was cross or did not like her. She would not want to elaborate on this but would switch to a dramatization in which she usually was the "boss," often demanding more play materials even when she had enough. At the end of the session she would again talk of her fear about what might happen the next day.

Helen seemed to bring her anxieties verbally at the beginning of each hour, then to defend against them by various dramatizations, ending the hour with another verbalized anxiety. Perhaps there is significance in the fact that Helen's defenses operated in this way. There might be transference implications in her expressing anxieties on coming and going and also in her being the boss in her dramatizations. The sequence of verbalizations and nonverbal activities may be significant, but little is known about the switching from one mode of expression to another. Therapists know most, perhaps, about the defensive aspects of such changes, but a change in the underlying content of the material may well be indicated not only by what is brought in but by the particular mode in which it is brought. This is relevant to the example of Ronald I., who was eleven years five months when treatment began, and thirteen years three months at the time of indexing:

After a series of short breaks in treatment Ronald began to act like a very small baby, using baby talk and sign language, expecting the therapist to understand his wishes and needs immediately and even to predict them in advance. "Poor Ronnie," he would say in a baby voice. He asked if I thought he would starve over the holiday break. In this way he introduced material which referred back to his separation from his mother when he was two years old.

Ronald's case illustrates a child's use of a mixture of modes of expression; although the child brought verbal material, his attitudes and demeanor indicated his wishes in a nonverbal fashion. The nonverbal mode of expression entailed a degree of regression; the child acted as if he were a baby again. The predominant mode of expression demonstrates the ways in which a particular child permits himself to remember important childhood events. Part of the ego must be available in order for the patient to comprehend what is going on when this behavior is interpreted. The effect of the relatively permissive atmosphere of the analytic situation should not be underestimated. Permissiveness allows subjects to come up which would have been more actively suppressed before. These subjects may show themselves in a variety of ways, not necessarily in the form of transference. The therapist's aim is to talk about these manifestations with the patient as much as possible.

Changes of material

Both regressive moves and forward moves are significant in child analysis. It is sometimes difficult, if not impossible, to know which changes are brought about by the analytic process and which by other factors. Development may be facilitated by any one of these other factors and by analysis. There can be changes due to the analytic process, to the situation in the child's environment outside analysis, and to development. Arousal of substantial anxiety or guilt in a

To Index: Describe shifts in the child's ways of bringing in material brought about during or by the analytic process. Watch for progressive moves, such as from gross bodily discharge to symbolic play, or from actions to verbalizations. In certain phases of treatment, watch for changes in the opposite direction, or regressive changes. If there is little or no change in the way in which the child brings up material in the course of analysis, comment on this fact.

child may lead to the use of gross bodily activities as modes of expression. Although a change to verbalization may be due to the child's progressive development, it is very often due to a reduction of anxiety or guilt. In the case of a child who threw things at his therapist while accusing him of being very "bad," the child was dealing with guilt feelings by identifying with an attacking and primitive superego figure. When this was interpreted and the child could see how he felt criticized internally, just as his mother still criticized him for many things, he quieted down. He was then able to discuss problems with the analyst which he could not discuss at the beginning of his analysis, when he had been able to use only nonverbal modes of expression or to shout abuse.

ANNA FREUD   One should not give too much credit to the analysis for changes in a child's mode of expression. Within a single session there may be a shift from baby talk to the verbal expression of fantasies, and back again, or such a shift may take place over a much longer period of time. The significance of such changes is different in each context. Changes in content, for example from pure fantasy to reality concerns, may sometimes be useful as indicators of therapeutic progress.

The cases of Andy V. and Norma Y. show changes in the ways in which material was brought during treatment. Andy was the younger of the two, beginning treatment at the age of two years six months, and indexed at three years two months:

At the beginning of treatment, material was brought in usually by enactment, such as hitting, kicking, biting, scratching, pinching, hugging, kissing, holding hands, sitting on the therapist's knee. Sometimes Andy would accompany these activities by pertinent verbalizations. At the beginning of the terminal phase of treatment, his communications became almost entirely verbal, especially those relating to his aggression. He was able to ask direct questions about termination.

Norma began treatment when she was four years eleven months old and was indexed when she was five years two months:

Norma was referred from nursery school because of excessive timidity and a pseudo-retardation of development. In the first weeks of treatment, she expressed her anxieties by diffuse aggressive activity—hurtling, splashing, hitting, biting, stamping, cutting—directed mostly at the play materials.

Later such behavior occurred only near the end of sessions, particularly by anal messing, expressing Norma's anger with the therapist. At times she played at being a "biting, scratching pussy-cat," thus attempting to distance herself from her aggressive impulses. By the end of the first year of analysis Norma's verbalized expression of anger became more frequent.

In both these children, the modes of expression changed because of the progress of the analysis that resulted from the analyst's verbal interventions. Since both children were very young, their ego development was undoubtedly another important factor in the changes. Changes may occur for a variety of reasons, but child therapists should keep in mind that the therapist's verbalizations may not have a direct connection with a conflict and nevertheless may still produce an effect on the patient's behavior. The therapist's incredulous repetition of something a patient has said may lessen the patient's conflict by indicating to him that an act he has spoken of was quite normal, or that the parents' behavior was abnormal, and the patient may feel a reduction of guilt or a lessening of some other conflict. Without mentioning the conflict directly the therapist's verbalization may have the effect of lessening it or helping to resolve it.

Norma's treatment provides a good example of the necessity to distinguish between regression as a result of the analytic process and an initial relaxation of restrictions as a consequence of the relatively permissive attitude in the playroom. The freedom of the analytic setting mobilized anxieties in Norma at the same time as it allowed her to relax some of the restrictions she placed on her impulses. As the analytic work progressed, Norma's expression of anger and rage increasingly took the form of an object-related anal attack, with a shift from direct expression in action, to play, and then to verbal expression.

In the case of Tommy E., a latency child, the reasons for changes in mode of expression were more limited. He was nine years seven months at the beginning of treatment and twelve years one month at the time of indexing:

When Tommy began treatment he played a variety of games with dreary regularity. On very rare occasions, he played imaginative or fantasy games. Although mostly defensive, these activities did enable Tommy to bring verbal material at times. Three years later, he mainly talked, but in periods of resistance he returned to his preoccupation with his school timetable or to beating out the rhythms of jazzy tunes.

Some of the change in Tommy E. between the ages of nine and twelve may be attributed to ego development, in that his way of playing changed from what was appropriate to a latency child to what was more appropriate to a twelve-year-old. Typical for a certain type of latency child were long periods of activities in the analysis serving defense and resistance. Tommy's behavior can thus be taken as reflecting a change in the nature of the play activities used as defenses, rather than as a change from one mode of expression to another.

Material on Frank O. illustrates changes due to the analytic work. Seven years seven months at the beginning of treatment, Frank was eight years eight months at the time of indexing:

At the beginning of treatment Frank spoke little but expressed his feelings by blushing and by various enactments, such as sitting close to the therapist. Negative feelings were expressed by throwing things at the therapist and by other forms of aggressive or messy play. He accepted and responded behaviorally to verbalizations by the therapist but did not take over the use of verbalization himself. Gradually more organized fantasy play developed, eventually accompanied by a running commentary. In this way his fantasy life unfolded and could be analyzed. Although he still blushed and used enactment to show positive feelings, Frank easily and spontaneously verbalized negative feelings toward the therapist.

Frank showed a change from using action to show his negative feelings to verbalizing them more easily and spontaneously. Although in his case there were in fact changes in his environment of some magnitude, it seems that much of the change was the result of the analytic work. The change did not interfere with Frank's capacity to play and his pleasure in playing, but it facilitated his ability to distinguish better between fantasy and reality.

13

Acting Out

Acting out is a clinical concept, not a metapsychological one. The enactment of wishes during a session, as by throwing things at the therapist or by seeking physical contact, is often called acting out, but the term should be limited to analytic material expressed in behavior outside the analytic setting. To include behavior both inside and outside the session, a more general term could be used, such as *enactment through motor means.* The classical view of the consequences of acting out for the analysis is that the impulses or feelings concerned are deflected from the therapist and from the analysis, and that by virtue of being expressed outside the treatment, they are not available for analytic work. To the degree that the treatment alliance and the self-observing functions are not interfered with, however, such material will be reported in the analytic sessions. Acting out does not necessarily mean the material is excluded from subsequent analysis.

A distinction should be made between acting out and the behavior of habitual "enactors" whose life-styles are characterized by their living out of impulses and wishes.

ANNA FREUD   Once I heard of the treatment of a woman who sought analysis because she kept getting pregnant. After a short period of analysis she told the therapist she was pregnant again. The therapist interpreted to her that she wanted a baby from him. I disagreed very much with the idea that this pregnancy represented a transference baby and also with calling the patient's behavior act-

---

To Index: Record instances of acting-out behavior stemming exclusively from the analytic work or related to the analytic process but occurring outside the session.

ing out. The woman had gotten pregnant repeatedly for years, and there was no evidence at all of a connection between the latest pregnancy and developments in the transference.

The question remains of how to understand "enacting," the living out of impulses and wishes, in children. Children, especially very young ones, act and enact within and outside the analytic situation, instead of just verbalizing. Therapists expect that the developing child will increasingly accompany enactments with verbalizations. A distinction can be made between this kind of normal enactment and so-called acting out in the transference: in the former, a wish or impulse is lived out with whoever is available at the moment. In the acting out in the transference, there is a return, in the course of and in consequence of the analytic work, of that which was repressed. A new derivative is formed which involves the specific person of the therapist. The derivative in turn is not permitted access to consciousness but is also repressed. It then finds a displaced expression outside the analysis involving a person other than the therapist. Instead of appearing within the session, this particular transference derivative is kept outside and "acted out" there.

The treatment of a preschool child, Greta F., illustrates the distinction between normal enactment and acting out in the transference. Greta was two years eight months old when treatment began and four years eight months at the time of indexing:

From the beginning of treatment Greta's behavior at home reflected her experiences in her sessions, whether these experiences were anxiety-arousing or anxiety-relieving. She frequently carried over material from sessions to the home to be "continued" there. In the first month of treatment, when the therapist interpreted her desire for a penis, she asked her father to get a hammer and screwdriver to mend her so that she could be a boy.

There are different ways of understanding Greta's material. It could well be that this very young child's behavior reflects the way in which children under age three understand, express, and react to the meaning of what is said to them.

ANNA FREUD   It is also possible that the verbal interpretation of the wish for a penis, given to a child of this age, can reinforce the existing wish for a penis and at the same time enhance the expectation that an adult can remedy the situation. Her behavior then appears to be entirely age-appropriate.

A further example comes later in Greta's treatment:

In the second year of treatment, Greta brought material showing her concern about the anal and aggressive aspects of her intercourse fantasies. The therapist reconstructed her fright and her soiling reactions on witnessing the parents having intercourse during the previous summer vacation. In response to this interpretation, Greta walked unobserved into her parents' bedroom that same night and witnessed sexual intercourse again. The parents reported this incident, adding that they did not know how long Greta had been watching.

Again, there are a number of possible ways of viewing Greta's material. The reconstruction of it by the therapist might have been incorrect, but the result of the intervention was that the child's sexual curiosity was further stimulated by the therapist's remarks. If the interpretation to Greta had been that she was very curious about her parents' sexual activities and that she wanted to see them, Greta's response could have been the consequence of taking the interpretation concretely as permission to act on her impulse. The example is more complicated, however, because the interpretation was formulated in terms of the child's anxiety, and her reaction to the intervention suggests several possibilities. She may have been attempting to master her anxiety and excitement in this situation now, or she may have wanted to reassess her perception of reality. Whatever the meaning of her reaction, neither of these two examples from Greta's treatment fits the definition of acting out as the expression of analytic material outside the analytic setting. Although Greta's behavior stemmed from the analytic work, it was developmentally appropriate for a child of this age to carry material freely from home to treatment and vice versa, to use the therapist and the parents interchangeably, and to employ a concrete mode of thinking. Hence the example is a poor one to illustrate acting out. It raises the important question of whether the concept of acting out is applicable in any way to very young children. It may well not be.

The latency child, Frank O., whose material was indexed when he was ten years one month old, two years and a half after treatment began, exhibited what seemed more like true acting out:

In the third year of his analysis, Frank enacted within the sessions fantasies of intercourse, pregnancy, and abortion, showing his wishes for the death of his infant sibling and his mother. He subsequently became very frightened and ran out of the session. He vomited on arriving home and complained of stomach ache. He was given aspirin at home, without relief. During the night he became "hysterical" with fear, rolling around the bed in pain and shouting, "I want to die," "I will do myself in." The general practitioner sent Frank straight to the hospital because of the possibility of acute appendicitis. The hospital found nothing physically abnormal, and Frank was sent home after three days. This was seen as the acting out of a childbirth fantasy and of his mother's suicide attempt, which had occurred before his younger brother was born. Frank later brought verbal confirmation of this interpretation in his analysis. It should be mentioned that his mother had deserted the family shortly after the baby was born.

Although there is a difference between acting out and hysterical conversion symptoms and somatizations, the term *acting out* can be used very broadly to describe Frank's behavior. In a general sense, the material of Frank's example fits the definition of acting out. Because the material emerging in the session aroused more anxiety than he could cope with in the analysis, Frank ran away from the session but enacted the material outside. If what was being enacted was the recovery of a memory, it is possible that had he not run away, the whole episode might have taken place within the session and been understood and interpreted by the therapist there, and hospitalization might have been avoided.

The question of why Frank ran out of the session can be answered in several ways. It may be only that his verbalizing his wishes for the death of his baby brother and his mother mobilized so much anxiety because of the mother's desertion. Or the experience may be understood in the context of the transference; for example, Frank's wishes for the death of the therapist-mother frightened him so much that he reversed the roles and acted out. Clearly in the enactment at home he identified with his perception of his mother. In leaving the session, he may have been running away from his impulses. He may have been running away from the therapist because he feared he would damage her. Or he may have been the mother deserting the therapist-child. The material in the example can be understood in several different ways.

Tina K. was an adolescent when she began treatment, aged sixteen years five months; indexing was done two years later:

Acting out of transference feelings occurred frequently during treatment. For example, when Tina was unable to bring her fears of being rejected by the therapist to the sessions, she provoked scenes at home with her mother in order to be rejected by her. Also, when defending against her homosexual wishes toward the therapist in the transference, Tina talked about her tender feelings for her mother and dressed seductively, wearing tight slacks and dark glasses.

Tina's homosexual acting out increased markedly after she moved out of the family home, and her homosexual transference intensified. Either her homosexual transference had become stronger, or her homosexuality had been "freed" and was being expressed now in a generalized way outside the analytic setting. All of the behavior in the example can be understood as a consequence of the tenuousness of the defenses at Tina's disposal.

Another example of acting out comes from the case of Katrina L., a latency child, who was six years one month old when treatment began, seven years one month old at the time of indexing:

From the time when Katrina's anal strivings manifested themselves more strongly in the treatment situation, she was prone to act out her anal impulses outside treatment, particularly at school, where together with other children she made up anal songs and verses, and called people "plops" and "poo-poo." After the summer vacation, Katrina's acting out became more and more directed against a new Indian teacher. She gave the teacher anal names and wrote anal slogans into her own books. Katrina also produced "books" whose content centered around bodily products such as feces and urine. Eventually Katrina, together with two other girls, had to see the headmistress because of the deprecatory remarks they had made about her teacher. Katrina was rather anxious about this visit even though she constantly denied her worry. In the working through of this material, Katrina wrote an anal story about the therapist, which was interpreted in the transference. After this the acting out lessened considerably and the anal material receded into the background.

Because Katrina's involvement with her Indian teacher seems to have foreshadowed the transference development, it might be viewed as an acting out of the transference. However, Katrina's behavior in fact illustrates a spilling over of the analytic situation, because the anal strivings were manifested more strongly in the treatment hour and then appeared outside treatment. If these impulses were to be acted out, they would have been manifested in behavior only outside treatment, rather than inside or both.

The unfolding of the anal fantasies in Katrina's case may be viewed more appropriately in the context of the analytic process. The analysis of defenses can lead to a general freeing up, both inside and outside the analysis, of impulses which had been kept back. The arrival of a brown-skinned teacher acted as an adventitious focus around which the anal impulses became more directly object-related, and the resulting conflicts were expressed in the transference and in the defenses against it. Acting out can thus be seen as a clinical concept closely linked with the idea of resistance to the analytic process, in particular resistance to emerging transference feelings.

The behavior of Jerry N., indexed when he was aged six years four months, two years after beginning treatment, is another example of acting out:

Jerry was not a child who used acting out a great deal. There was some slight tendency to act out his aggression toward his sister at home when he and his therapist were discussing his sibling jealousy early in analysis. A rather more noticeable instance of acting out came when he reacted to interpretations of his sadistic intercourse fantasies with a great deal of anxiety. This led to his making an announcement in public, to his parents' great embarrassment, that his therapist had said mommies and daddies hurt each other in bed. He afterward told the therapist about this incident and threatened her with his mother's anger should she ever refer to the subject again. When the therapist discussed his acting out with him, he simply said he would repeat it in order to stop her talking about it. His mother had helped reduce acting out to a minimum by always telling him immediately that his analysis was the place for such behavior and he should reserve it for his sessions.

Clearly, acting out was linked in Jerry's case with impulsive activity by a rather young child. Hence the attack on Jerry's sibling is another instance of spillover. In child analysis therapists frequently see a reaction to interpretation which suggests that the intervention has given the child license to enact a well-defended-against wish. Jerry's use of his parents to blackmail the therapist into silence may have been an attempt to deal with the anxiety mobilized by interpretations. This anxiety spilled over and led to his making the public announcement about adult sexual behavior.

Although some analysts define acting out rather narrowly, the term is used in work with children in a relatively broad sense. It is used to describe any expression by the child of unconscious material which the therapist would prefer to see in the form of fantasy or other verbal material brought within the analysis, preferably linked with the transference. Three more subdivisions of this broad concept of acting out can be derived from clinical material. First, it may include a spilling over of analytic material, including the transfer from the sessions to life outside the treatment. Material that is enacted outside the analytic sessions stems from the analytic work and from the loosening of defenses. Very young children, like Greta F., who go to their parents for confirmation and gratification, provide frequent examples of this behavior. Katrina L.'s material also illustrates spillover. Second, it may represent the expression in action of past memories which have been revived. An enactment in a setting outside the analytic situation, like Frank O.'s apparent appendicitis attack, may occur. Finally, it may be an acting out in the transference. Acting out for defensive reasons is exemplified by Tina K.'s behavior, as well as by Katrina L.'s involvement with her Indian teacher.

14

Coming and Going

The therapist usually accompanies children to and from the waiting room. This aspect of the therapist's contact with the child may, in certain cases and at certain times, have special significance for the treatment. For some children, especially little ones, entering through the doors of a psychoanalytic clinic or office represents the beginning of the session, while for others the session begins when the therapist appears. There are some patients who, on arriving, run to the treatment room whether or not the therapist is available. Others are reluctant to enter the waiting room and may roam the halls, whereas still others keep the therapist waiting. When time comes to end the session, some children have difficulty in leaving, whereas others run out early. If there is a long distance to walk from the waiting room to the treatment room, a child of any age may use the opportunity to bring up material outside the treatment room.

ANNA FREUD   The waiting room is a place where the mother and therapist often meet. There are some children who want such a meeting to happen, whereas others seek to prevent it. Many children have mixed feelings about it. The child's motivations may vary too. For example, a child may want to keep the therapist for himself, or he may be caught in a loyalty conflict over his feelings about his therapist and his parents.

To Index: Record significant events between the time of the child's arrival at the place of treatment and the beginning of the session, or at the end of sessions between leaving the treatment room and leaving the vicinity of the building. Note special features (e.g. difficulty in leaving, enactment or play on the stairs). Record the form of the behavior, how it is understood, the technical handling of the situation, and the way the situation was utilized in the analytic work.

What goes on in the waiting room often affects a child's behavior. If the waiting room is a busy place, children see other patients and their families, which influences some children to a significant degree. It also affects the material brought to the session. Therapists occasionally forget how much events and experiences in the waiting room can affect the immediate material brought by the child, who may make no direct reference to what has happened in the waiting room but may nevertheless be profoundly influenced by what has occurred.

Technical problems concerning waiting situations with children contrast with problems arising with adults. The beginnings and endings of sessions are necessarily more flexible for children. Getting the child to the treatment room may require giving interpretations in the waiting room or on the stairs. Because she is within earshot of others, the therapist may phrase such interpretations differently from the way she would phrase them in the treatment room; thus the therapist's experience, embarrassment, or concern for the patient's privacy influence what she says. These considerations apply equally on leaving the treatment room and going to the waiting room.

In principle, therapists aim to do analytic work with children in the consulting room just as in adult analysis, although with many children this takes time to achieve and requires a degree of flexibility in the child therapist.

Ronald I. was one of those children who wait until they are in the treatment room before beginning their session, and therefore his therapist might have expected that he would not present a technical problem. He was eleven years five months when treatment began and thirteen years three months when the indexing was done:

Ronald was always charming, poised, well-mannered, and polite on entering and leaving the clinic. This was in marked contrast to his behavior within the treatment room, where he was teasing, rude, babyish, and aggressive. The contrast paralleled his charming behavior outside the home and his infantile and aggressive behavior within the family.

The therapist who observes a change of behavior between waiting room and treatment room, or whose attention is drawn to it, may be able to utilize the information in the analytic work, especially if it is known to parallel other changes, as in Ronald's case.

Behavior on coming and going in a much younger child is illus-

trated by Andy V., who was indexed when he was three years two
months old, eight months after his treatment began:

The general pattern was for Andy to start the session on the stairs with play
and fantasies. He wanted to hold the therapist's hand. At one stage he
crawled upstairs on hands and knees, asking to be carried. The crawling
stopped when it was interpreted as his wish to be a little baby. During the
same period he had various methods of coming downstairs—on his knees,
on his back, on his front. This behavior was provocative and was concurrent
with provocative behavior at home. It invited smacking as a means of controlling his aggression and as part of his intercourse fantasies. On leaving
sessions he sometimes played a hiding and finding game, running away
from the therapist to hide behind a coat hanging on one of the landings. He
screamed with delight on being found. This was seen as an acting out of the
anticipated reunion with the therapist the following day, a means of controlling his anxiety about separating. When he met staff members on his way to
and from the session, he was frequently aggressive toward them, calling
them "Mrs. Bum" or "fuckie bogies." He often "shot" the males he met.
When a certain point in his positive relationship with the therapist had been
reached, he would hold the therapist's hand on going downstairs and then
launch himself into space.

Andy V. illustrates the range of behavior a two-and-one-half-
year-old can display on coming and going. It is to be expected that a
child of this age will begin the session when the therapist appears.
Nevertheless, some therapists do try to discourage this; to children
who begin to enact or express themselves on the stairs, for example,
they may suggest that the treatment room is a more appropriate
place. Many factors have to be considered, such as the age-appropriateness of the behavior, the total setting at the time, and the possible
meanings of the material for the analytic work with a particular
child.

Behavior around the ending of a session can be significant. Jerry
N. began treatment at four years four months, and the indexing was
at six years four months:

Jerry always attempted to control the ending of the sessions. Early in treatment he reacted badly to ending sessions. This was linked with his separation anxieties and the fear that the therapist might not come back the next
day. The therapist took to warning him a little before the end of a session.
He then accepted the ending of sessions better, but he himself had to decide
when the time was up. Gradually he came to judge how much time he had
left, was usually accurate when he announced that the time was up, and felt
more comfortable being in control in this way.

ANNA FREUD   I have found that behavior such as shown in this example is quite common in child analysis. It is by no means restricted to those children who have a need to control the adult. There are many factors to be considered, such as the child's immature capacity to judge time.

A young child may not grasp the rationale for limiting the time of sessions, although he may eventually learn to accept the routine. Naturally children, like adults, resent being suddenly interrupted in their activities.

Some children spontaneously participate in tidying up toys or cleaning up a mess in the treatment room. Others habitually dissociate themselves from such tasks. Some therapists intervene and attempt to get the child's cooperation, reasoning that this demonstrates that analysis is a joint effort. For many children the clearing up process represents a sealing over of regressed fantasy material that has emerged in the sessions. If a therapist wishes to encourage this sealing over process, asking the child to help with tidying up at the end of the sessions may help. Each patient can utilize the ending of sessions to express a variety of problems. Every child therapist is familiar with the patient who angrily makes a mess just before departing and with the patient who repeats the battle over toilet training in regard to clearing up after the session.

The treatment of Dorothy J. demonstrates what can be called "role playing" on coming and going. Dorothy was three years nine months old when treatment began; the indexing was done when she was five years five months old:

For a period of several months Dorothy insisted that she and the therapist adopt fantasy roles and speak only in character while going to and from the sessions. For example, Dorothy adopted the role of "big school girl" and told off the "little girl therapist" for some pretended misdemeanor. Similarly, on leaving the session, Dorothy pretended she was a "big school girl" monitor leading the way out of school. This behavior was understood and interpreted as a defense against experiencing and expressing anger toward the persons from whom she had to separate, especially the mother and the therapist.

The behavior of Dorothy J. is an interesting demonstration of a reversal of roles reserved for going up and down the stairs on the way to the treatment room. The child may have attached some special significance to the stairs on the basis of experiences at school, but her therapist was quite sure that the behavior related specifically to the transition from mother to therapist, and to the feelings which this event aroused. Behavior on coming and going may be intimately involved with the patient's symptomatology, as in the case of a little boy referred for treatment because of his fear of going up stairs. His therapist's treatment room was several flights up, on the top floor. It took the child a half-hour to reach the treatment room, as he had to struggle to overcome his fear every day. Perhaps the progress of the analysis would have been different if the child had been treated on the ground floor.

Adolescent patients too display various types of behavior in coming to and going from sessions, as did Charles Z., eleven years four months old when treatment began, and fourteen years one month at the time of this indexing:

Even in his third year of treatment Charles still refused to use the waiting room. If it was necessary for him to wait, he sat on the landing outside the treatment room. This was at first interpreted as his wish to be in control and his difficulty in sharing. By the end of the third year, however, Charles was able to talk about the feelings of shyness and embarrassment he experienced if he went into the waiting room. He did not like "to be looked at." This was linked with his general manner on coming to the clinic: he dashed upstairs, frowning and avoiding other people's eyes or greetings.

It took Charles' therapist a long time to understand that his avoidance of the waiting room was not his wish to be in control but rather a reflection of his embarrassment at having to wait there for the therapist. His fantasies about the waiting room needed to be known in order for his behavior to be understood fully.

Michael B. was seven years eight months when this material was recorded, a year and ten months after his analysis began:

Throughout his analysis Michael insisted on having a ritual "two kisses" on parting from his father at the clinic when he was brought each morning. When he did not receive these kisses, he became agitated, and in the end his father would provide the "magic"; thus he was forgiven his hostile wishes to the father. When the therapist asked him what he thought would happen if his father kissed him only once or three times, Michael replied, "My penis would fall off. My biggest worry is that my penis-bottom will break."

The adolescent patient Tina K. had been in analysis for two years and was eighteen and one-half years old when this excerpt was recorded:

Especially at the beginning of treatment, Tina used to tiptoe into the clinic, hardly pressing the bell of the door; she carried a parcel of high-heeled shoes to wear for her session. She took a very long time in the cloakroom to wash and to make herself up. In the waiting room, her artificial "ladylike" behavior provoked attention and interest. At some periods in her analysis, Tina spent over an hour in the waiting room before or after the session in order to be able to make closer observations of the therapist's activities in the clinic.

Behavior on coming to and going from the session is an important area of observation. It can be extremely meaningful, giving the therapist insight into aspects of the patient's functioning which might not be available within the treatment room, but it can also be a source of technical difficulty. Many therapists are uncomfortable about their interaction with their patients before and after sessions, or uncomfortable about reporting this interaction. Nevertheless, the child's behavior and interaction with the therapist are of the greatest relevance to child analytic technique.

Part Four

Interpretation
and
Intervention

15

Introducing Treatment

Therapists vary in the ways they introduce the child to analysis, in regard to both the idea of treatment and its method. The way in which the therapist goes about introducing the child to the idea or even to the technique of treatment depends to some extent on whether the child herself wants help or is suffering from worries and anxieties, or whether she denies or is oblivious of her own disturbance. It may not be easy to determine at the outset what the patient's real attitudes to treatment are. An initial apparently cooperative and understanding attitude may be followed by strong resistances which make analysis difficult. Conversely, a patient who is silent at the beginning may very well have a real wish for or expectation of getting help from the treatment. A treatment alliance is something that develops over time on the basis of the patient's growing positive attachment to the therapist and increasing awareness of her own need for help, neither of which may be present at the outset.

There are differences between introducing the child to the aims or purpose of treatment and acquainting the child with the method of treatment. It is often easier for younger children to understand that treatment has something to do with getting help than it is to grasp why there are certain rules about treatment. A boy of four and one-half years was told that he was being brought to analysis so that he and his mother would not fight so much. He answered that he liked

To Index: Record how treatment is introduced to the child, including how the reasons for and the methods of the analysis are presented to the child. Note the child's reactions. Focus on the therapist's interventions, including the handling of what the child has heard about therapy from other people, e.g. his mother.

fighting with his mommy. This child's therapist was faced with the task of helping the child to deal with a problem which reflected his own and his mother's pathology. The boy might have been quite prepared to come in order to play, but he now saw no further reason for coming, though he was willing to cooperate with the "method."

Another boy, of eight, reported in the first session that his severe tics had completely cleared up. He coped with his anxiety during the first few sessions by expressing pleasure in having someone with whom to play cards. He said, "Now I see why I come to play with you. It takes my mind off my worries." This child's anxieties led him to use the treatment situation defensively. There is no formula about how to introduce a child to treatment. In fact, a standardized format for handling initial sessions, without regard to the nature of the child's disturbance or the degree of his awareness of it, may well interfere with the optimal development of the analytic work.

Kenny K. had been in treatment three years and was nine years three months old when this material was indexed:

Kenny seemed to be pleased to come to the clinic since he had worried about his soiling and had been increasingly constipated. The mother had introduced the idea of treatment as Kenny's "going to see a man who could help him with his worries about his poos." In the first week of treatment, Kenny echoed this view, saying that the therapist was interested in Kenny's poos. The therapist consistently made the point that he was there to help with any worries about which Kenny might need help. The therapeutic situation was readily linked to his sadomasochistic problems as they found expression in his everyday life and in the transference. The analysis gradually seemed to become a valuable part of Kenny's attempt to find solutions to fears and reality problems such as separations, abandonment, punishment, exclusion, ridicule, body damage, and anatomical differences. Yet when Kenny first voluntarily brought up his "worries" over his poos in the second year of treatment, he referred to everything that had gone before as "play." This was understood by the therapist as Kenny's way of saying that he had repeated with the therapist his sadomasochistic interplay with his mother.

It is possible that Kenny's analysis would have been facilitated if his soiling symptom had been taken up directly from the beginning. The mother's collusion with the child's soiling later seemed to be repeated by the patient in the transference. By not referring to the soiling for a long time, the therapist may have played his countertransference part in the collusion. Naturally it is difficult to know at the outset of analysis the significance to the patient of the presenting symptoms. When Kenny echoed his mother's statement that his soiling was the reason he was coming to treatment, he might have been expressing either an excessive anxiety about his symptom or an excitement with which he hoped to involve the therapist. In either case, there may have been justification for the therapist to respond in the way he did.

ANNA FREUD   Early in the history of psychoanalytic technique it was considered important not to focus on symptoms as such, because they were thought to be no more than compromise formations appearing on the surface. In adult analysis there are techniques which bring up from the depths of the mind those conflicting forces which underlie the symptoms. Child analysis does not have such techniques so readily available, for analysts cannot rely on free association. Therefore it is more important for the child analyst to make reference to the symptom in working with the child. For example, this may be done by an occasional remark, such as, "So that's why you have to behave so curiously about your constipation" or "Perhaps this fear we are discussing now is connected with why you can't go to the toilet," or "This is connected with why you have to upset your parents." There are certainly many references of this kind in Kenny's early material, but if the therapist leaves out what this all leads to, the child will be very glad to leave it out too. The therapist did not take up the child's initial remarks about his soiling and, more important, did not talk about it for a long time. Probably he was waiting for the child to talk about it again, but the child did bring it up, by soiling in the sessions.

Edward G. exemplifies the special situation of a child who is already familiar with the clinic where he is undergoing analysis and with some of the personnel, having attended other departments of the clinic before the beginning of treatment. Edward was three years one month old at the beginning of treatment and was indexed at the age of four years eleven months:

Edward had met the therapist twice before treatment began, since he had to accompany his mother to her preliminary interviews, being unable to separate. On these occasions, he heard his mother talking about the symptoms for which he was referred. As he had been told little about treatment, except that it was to help him with worries, he watched the therapist cautiously in these two interviews, gradually beginning to make tentative approaches to her; but first he needed his mother's permission, as it were. He would first try out a remark on his mother, then address the therapist. During the first week of treatment, he asked many questions about how the clinic differed from the well baby clinic and the nursery school. When the therapist explained that children sometimes had worries which they could not manage alone and that they sometimes needed special help, Edward nodded solemnly and said, "They do worry, children, sometimes." In the second week his fear that treatment might be a punishment and that the therapist might send him away for being naughty was brought out through stories of "Tom, Tom, the piper's son" and of the toy trains in Battersea Park on which only children were sent. When his fear of being sent away was taken up, he asked, "Does Miss A. [the therapist] send children away?" He was given reassurance that the therapist was there to understand things, not to punish him.

Perhaps at the beginning of treatment, such a young child cannot really have any idea of the purpose of treatment. To a child, analysis probably seems simply to be another one of those strange activities that grown-ups enter into with children and which children cannot yet understand but simply accept, responding to whatever is put to them. The child's experience in treatment gradually enables him to sort out the meaningful differences between the treatment situation and other situations in his life. This is part of his task of adaptation, even if he speaks of treatment as "play." Hence an intellectual explanation of the purpose of treatment is probably of little value, other than to reassure the child about his initial anxieties and expectations about treatment, as was probably the intention of the therapist in Edward's case.

Therapists have different ways of introducing children to treatment. Some always begin the first session by explaining to the child the circumstances, the frequency of attendance, and the purpose of treatment. Others do not make such a deliberate introduction but, as Edward's therapist did, listen to what the child says, pick up the child's anxieties and fantasies about treatment, and interpret them. How the introduction is handled depends on the therapist's perception of the patient's defenses and the nature of the child's anxieties, so a formula is inappropriate. Both styles of introducing the child to treatment are affected by whether or not a previous diagnostic evaluation was done and by whom and whether any explanation of treatment was offered to the child at that stage.

Esther L., aged eight years ten months at the time, was given an explanation of treatment by her mother when it was begun; the indexing was done a year later:

Her mother tried to prepare Esther for treatment by saying that it was to help her because she was often unhappy, worried about school, and found difficulties in making friends. Esther denied having any problems when the therapist tried to discuss her reasons for coming to the clinic and how treatment worked. In view of her strong defenses, especially denial, the therapist could only gradually take up the various problems that brought her to treatment. Esther's attitude was to brush aside these topics, withdraw into silence, or change the subject.

ANNA FREUD   The analyst understood that Esther's strong defenses reflected her intense anxiety about what would happen to her in treatment. No introduction could be of any use to her until she developed a relationship to the analyst which allowed the analyst to take up the child's defenses.

An essential element in introducing a child to treatment is making contact with the patient and his problem. If this can be done, the patient will feel he can be understood and the idea of treatment may then make sense to him. It is important that the therapist always say that she is there to help the child with his worries. Even if the child does not respond to the reassurance immediately, putting this stance into words helps to structure the therapeutic situation.

16

Clarification and Confrontation

What is meant or understood by the term *interpretation* is not always clear and is certainly controversial. The therapist does all sorts of things to help the patient make conscious what is unconscious, and to prepare him to accept things which he could not accept previously. In child analysis, the therapist often precedes or accompanies the work of interpretation by clarifying or explaining certain internal or external events and processes to the child. These verbal interventions pave the way for interpretations, or in some way supplement interpretations. It is sometimes necessary to help the child distinguish between fantasy and reality, to give other factual information, or to provide reassurance. In this context reassurance means only explanations of reality that are aimed at dispelling anxieties.

A magical quality is often attributed to an interpretation which seems to have led to some dramatic or noteworthy change in the patient. Close examination frequently reveals that a great deal of preparatory work has been done beforehand, so that defining interpretation on the basis of its effectiveness alone is misleading.

ANNA FREUD   One should distinguish between the interpretation of content and the interpretation of defense. It is an old question— whether the interpretation of a defense really has the same quality as an interpretation of unconscious content. In making a patient aware of a defense, the analyst is drawing the patient's attention to an automatic process which was not unconscious in the metapsy-

To Index: Give examples of instances when clarification, explanation, or reassurance is of special importance in the case, and why.

chological sense. This allows the analyst to approach the content, that which is defended against, more gradually.

One view has it that an interpretation is a statement which includes the relationship between the defense and what is defended against, which is often made in a number of stages, and which makes the patient aware of something of which he was previously unaware. But this is probably too narrow a view of interpretation.

Susan S., aged three years one month at the beginning of treatment, suffered from constitutional sexual precocity, for which she had been hospitalized at the age of twenty months; her case was indexed when she was six years six months:

After Susan had enumerated the reasons that various members of her family had been in the hospital, the therapist broached the subject of her hospitalization at twenty months, about which Susan had heard many confusing accounts. She asked the therapist to tell her why she had been in the hospital then. The therapist complied with Susan's request, as she felt it would help Susan to know that her abnormality could be discussed on a reality level. She explained to Susan that her mommy had been worried because she was growing very fast and took her to the hospital to find out why. There they told her that she was a rather special baby. She grew faster than other children. She was ahead of them at the moment, but in time they would catch up with her, and then she would be like the other girls. Susan listened with rapt attention and asked the therapist to repeat it all over again. She then gave the therapist a present, drawing a picture of an Easter egg for her.

By explaining reality to Susan before exploring her fantasies, the therapist implied that Susan was confused because no one had ever explained her unusual body to her. The therapist thought that beginning work by talking about reality would make treatment possible. Thus she did not give an interpretation at this point but an explanation of reality, which was presumably also a reassurance. Susan was not prevented by this from bringing her own view of the reality and of her chaotic sexual fantasy life. Certainly some explanation and clarification of reality are essential in the treatment of children with significant physical handicaps. A similar approach may well be indicated when the child's parents are seriously disturbed emotionally. Unless the disturbance is discussed openly with the child, the analysis may founder. The child often has strong defenses against such material and may blame himself for whatever has gone wrong or may identify with the disturbed parents. It is often up to the analyst to initiate the discussion of the topic in order to clarify it.

Confrontation occurred in the treatment of Tommy E., who began treatment aged nine years seven months and whose material was indexed when he was twelve years one month old:

On two occasions, Tommy's analysis became blocked due to his inability to talk about quarrels between his parents. The therapist confronted Tommy with information given by the mother about the disharmony between her and her husband. It was taken up with Tommy in terms of his loyalty conflict, and he reacted with relief. He was then willing to talk about the quarrels at home and to bring his feelings about the quarrels into treatment.

The way Tommy's analyst handled the block raises the question whether a therapist is entitled to use information from an extra-analytic source. In this instance, however, what is described is not really giving the patient information, but rather making known to the patient that the therapist knows what the patient really knows. This might be called confrontation. When the child therapist is in contact with the parents, she at times has extra-analytic information which may help her to understand aspects of the patient's material more clearly, but which poses the technical problems of whether and how to use it.

Confrontation is not restricted to situations concerned with information from extra-analytic sources. At times, as when resistance to treatment is manifested by very irregular attendance, the patient and the parents may have to be told the conditions necessary for the continuation of the analysis. This approach may have to be resorted to either when the analysis of the resistance has failed or when the parents collude with the resistance.

Sexual information may have to be given to a patient, as it was to Jerry N., who began treatment at the age of four years four months and whose case was indexed when he was six years four months old:

Jerry brought many confused sexual fantasies and questions. Central to his concerns was the question of how babies are made. The therapist first analyzed the intercourse fantasies Jerry brought and later gave specific information about intercourse and birth when the child asked for it.

Unlike the case of the sexually precocious little girl, Susan S., who was given concrete information in response to questions before the fantasies were analyzed because, apparently, her therapist felt that the progress of the analysis depended on this information being given first, Jerry's case entailed no such requirement. Certainly the demand for information can be a resistance to, among other things, revealing specific fantasies. Even so, it may be more appropriate at a certain point to treat a question as a question and to answer it. Comments that facilitate interpretation are very important, as most of the interventions made by therapists are interpretations rather than explanations. The extent of the explanation required depends on the age of the child; the younger the child, the greater the need for explanation.

Information was given at first to Frank O., who was seven years seven months at the start of treatment and eight years eight months at the indexing:

At the beginning of treatment Frank appeared to have a poor ability to appraise reality and a tendency to withdraw into fantasy, as well as an insatiable wish to be taken care of by the therapist. Therefore, during the first six months of treatment, the therapist tended to give reality answers to Frank's questions, such as personal information about the therapist, rather than pursuing his fantasies. Subsequently a gradual changeover was made to the giving of interpretations as well as reality information, and by the eighth or ninth month of treatment interpretations predominated.

The reason for giving information in Frank's case seems to have been to establish and maintain the treatment relationship. There are certain disadvantages to this approach. The child may experience some inhibition of fantasying about the therapist as a consequence of the intervention or, at least, some inhibition in regard to bringing such fantasies to the analysis. By becoming too much of a real object for the child, the therapist may make the development of the transference more difficult to recognize or may interfere with it.

Katrina L.'s therapist felt that interpretations were not effective in relieving the child's anxiety, and so gave her reassurance. Katrina was six years one month old at the beginning of treatment; her case was indexed a year later:

During the early weeks of treatment Katrina was very much concerned whether things in her locker were safe. Similarly she was apprehensive that other people might interrupt her sessions whenever she heard footsteps on the stairs or children's voices outside. In addition to interpretations, the therapist repeatedly gave Katrina reassurances in order to reduce her anxieties in connection with these events. In spite of interpretations pertaining to loyalty conflicts and guilt feelings, Katrina remained anxious throughout the first year of treatment about the confidentiality of the treatment situation. Although the reassurances given allowed Katrina to gain greater confidence in the treatment, some fears and suspicions remained, as was gathered from her occasional remark that the therapist was a "nosy parker."

For Katrina, interpretation seemed to be inadequate in some way, and the child appeared to be in need of continual reassurance. Her fear of having her secret thoughts revealed to her parents may have covered yet another anxiety about revealing her secrets to the analyst. There does seem to be justification for reassuring a child about the confidentiality of treatment, especially in regard to clarifying for the child the therapist's role vis-à-vis the patient and the parents.

Another form of reassurance is to tell the child such things as, "I'm not going to let you do damaging things." Statements of this kind may be appropriate following an interpretation of a hostile or destructive wish or enactment, because it is quite common in child analysis for interpretation of a wish to be followed by its more direct expression and by an increase in the child's anxiety. The therapist may have to create a situation of containment and safety for the child before analyzing the accompanying anxiety. This applies particularly to very young children who still depend on the mother for external controls.

Anna Freud has pointed out that the analytic situation can be anxiety-arousing as well as anxiety-relieving, and she suggests that the various roles in which the therapist is cast—for example as seducer, auxiliary ego, superego—all reveal what the analytic situation represents to a child at that stage in his treatment. For many children, the analytic hour provides an enormous relief because the ego no longer feels so compelled to hide what goes on internally.

ANNA FREUD   I remember my very first child patient, who was an obsessional little girl under impossible pressure in her life to keep control of her various impulses. Once she said quite openly, "My only rest hour is the analytic hour."

Besides verbal reassurance, the therapist may offer nonverbal forms of reassurance. These may be expressed by physical contact, as by holding the child so he does not hit the therapist or by comforting the child on the therapist's lap. A criterion for the therapist's interventions is whether they promote or interfere with the analytic work. At times interpretations themselves appear to interfere with the work, as when some children react to all interpretations as attacks or criticisms and feel they must fight them off. Despite difficulties in this situation for the therapist, there are ways in which the interpretation can be given. It may be necessary to focus on the meaning to a child of being given an interpretation, whatever the content. At other times the impact of an interpretation might be softened without reducing its effectiveness by saying, for example, "I know this may make you angry, but . . ."

The therapist must remember that, however useful, clarifications, confrontations, and reassurances are just adjuncts to interpretation. The case material illustrates interventions which may have been useful in aiding the analysis proper to continue at a particular point; yet for the analysis to continue, appropriate interpretations must be given.

17

Aids to Interpretation

In child therapy toys, stories, dolls, role play, and various verbal devices are sometimes used in different ways to prepare the way for interpretation or to facilitate it. A common feature in these techniques is that they permit a degree of displacement or externalization of self and object representations and of the interaction between them. This displacement takes place onto other people or characters.

It is usually the child who initiates the use of play material in a way which reveals something about himself. The child may do this by choosing to play or work with an animal or a puppet or by telling a story. The therapist may then follow the child's lead and enter into the game, giving an interpretation in the form of a comment made by one of the toy figures or characters in the story, thus using the play character as a proxy. Usually the therapist couches her interpretation in terms of the toy or the character representing the child. Some children accept interpretations more easily when the interpretation does not refer directly to themselves but rather to another child, a puppet, a doll, or some character in a story.

Referring to other children is often a useful way of phrasing an interpretation. A therapist might say, "I once knew a child who always felt worried whenever he was angry with his mommy or daddy." However, some children cannot tolerate this method for a variety of reasons. It may arouse jealousy, or it may threaten the

To Index: Give examples of various techniques used to prepare the ground for or to facilitate interpretations (e.g., the use of stories, puppets). Note the extent to which these aids are used, whether they are used throughout the treatment or at particular points, and how the child responds.

child's self-esteem if he believes himself to be compared with other children.

The therapist must be careful not to collude too much with the child's defenses rather than analyzing them. If the child does not tolerate direct interpretations well, perhaps the defensive use of displacement should be analyzed by pointing out that the child would rather talk about someone else's problems than concentrate on those of his own. Anna Freud has pointed out that the procedure of giving interpretations about a person or figure onto whom the child has externalized aspects of his own self, thus accepting the externalization for the time being, is not necessarily collusion but, rather, a way of approaching threatening mental content gradually. The therapist may also use the technique of referring to a "part" of the child, saying, for example, "I think a part of you doesn't like to know about the angry thoughts inside you," in order to bring about in the child a greater awareness of his conflicts. Another and similar device is to "divide" the child into the "big boy" and the "little boy" who look at things differently. These techniques are all legitimate aids to interpretation which are used as steps in the analytic procedure.

ANNA FREUD   There are other features of a child's personality which enter into the readiness to make displacements and externalizations. It is very much easier for the child to criticize somebody else than to criticize himself. Very often such things as cleanliness or anything else that the child acquires gradually begins by the child criticizing another person. A good example is the young child who points with disgust and disapproval at another child wetting the floor, before he himself has attained sphincter control. I think this readiness to externalize and displace accounts for the fact that the existence of internal conflict is only very gradually accepted by the child in the course of the analytic work.

Michael B., seven years eight months old, had been in treatment for nearly two years at the time of the indexing:

Michael's first therapist invented an imaginary boy called Freddy in interpretative stories. In this guise Michael could accept interpretations which otherwise would have overwhelmed him. His second therapist felt it useful to introduce another boy, called Peter, who embodied changes resulting from the analytic work, as well as certain external changes. For example, Peter had different worries and a larger family, and a better ego than Michael. Another aid to interpretation which was useful at times when direct interpretation threatened to overwhelm Michael was telling picture stories (arranging pictures in a sequence so that they tell a story). This involved Michael in deciphering the interpretative material. He also responded to the use of drawings to represent his anxieties. Under these circumstances he could accept the interpretations which were pertinent to the situation.

Arranging pictures in rebus stories may work to further the analytic process by diminishing the child's shame or humiliation at being told something painful. By enlisting the active participation of the patient—for example, by having the patient work on a rebus story or by asking him what he makes of the story—the therapist can often help him to come to the answer himself, which increases his self-esteem and allows him to gain a feeling of mastery. Such techniques may be outgrown or become obsolete in the course of a particular treatment, without their use ever having to be analyzed.

Robert P. began treatment at the age of nine years eight months; his material was indexed when he was eleven years four months:

The therapist found that, in sessions during which Robert showed resistance, it was sometimes possible to reach him in various ways. Among these were using wit or entering a play situation, such as talking to Robert on a "pretend" phone and giving interpretations in this role.

A child may find it easier to begin to discuss difficult topics when the therapist offers opportunities for the patient to distance himself from the material at first.

Material from the treatment of Ilse T. was indexed when she was six years six months old, after one year and seven months of treatment:

Early in treatment Ilse expressed concern that being sent to treatment was a first step to being sent away from home. She brought up this material through role play in which the therapist was cast as Ilse and sent to a "lonely school," where she was to stay for the night. Rather than directly interpreting the content, the therapist, in her role as Ilse, complained of being sent to the clinic while her younger brother was at home with mommy. In the next role playing, Ilse as "teacher" developed a sympathetic attitude to the therapist as her "pupil." During that play she remarked spontaneously that she was not asking for mommy. Whereas this approach seemed to establish contact initially and to give Ilse the feeling that she was understood, it soon became necessary to abstain from entering into these dramatizations because Ilse began to utilize them for the purpose of denial. As "mother," Ilse would say, "Everyone is naughty; even I am," in order to deny her anxiety that she would be sent away from home as a punishment. She would also, in the role of mother, claim that she loved her daughter more than she did her baby son. In this way Ilse denied her feeling that the opposite was true.

In Ilse's example the role play was initiated by the child and entered into by the therapist, who reflected some of the child's current feelings about coming to treatment. Children often specify the role in which they cast the therapist, which helps the therapist understand the child's fantasies. In Ilse's case role assignment was an aid to understanding but also an aid to interpretation. But playing roles has its dangers, one of which is provoking resistance. The child may be offended and feel laughed at, or the child's loyalty to the mother may be challenged by what she feels is the therapist's ridicule of the mother. In a very young child reality testing may be undermined if the therapist enters too wholeheartedly into the dramatization. In choosing such an aid to interpretation and deciding to what extent to enter into it, the therapist should take into account the child's mode of expression and the child's need to defend himself.

Lydia S. began treatment at the age of five years seven months; her material was indexed when she was eight years old:

Lydia enacted her intense wishful fantasy life at home and in treatment almost from the start. Because Lydia's ego was so overwhelmed by her excitement, direct interpretation of her wishes was substituted for by attempts at containment by the therapist offering more "distanced" approaches, as in drawings or through interpretative stories about other people. Although Lydia knew that the people in these stories represented herself and her family, she could not accept interpretation in any other form.

A number of factors may account for the fact that telling interpretative stories often makes the essential content of the interpretation more acceptable to a child patient. In Lydia's case the associated affects may have been distanced by her drawing rather than by talking; or the interpretative stories may have been made acceptable to Lydia because the intensity of her guilt feelings was reduced by hearing that other people had similar problems.

Katrina L. had been in treatment one year when her case was indexed when she was seven years one month old:

At the beginning of treatment, it was found necessary to use stories concerning other children, because direct interpretations evoked considerable anxiety and aggression. Within some months Katrina came to recognize the "disguise" and tried to stop the therapist speaking whenever he embarked on a story about another child. After about a year, Katrina brought her own dressing-up dolls as substitute objects with which she could freely express her own wishes and feelings and which were also used as a helpful tool in the therapist's interpretations.

There is a danger that aids to interpretation can be overused or can come to be used routinely. Ideally they should be used or dropped according to the needs of the analytic situation. An example of what may happen with the overuse of such a technique is the case of a child who was given many interpretations about his friends. This simply established for him the feeling that criticism directed outward was permissible and that he was safe as long as others were being attacked.

ANNA FREUD   With all these aids to interpretation, it is important that the therapist and the child are together in understanding who is being talked about. There are some children whose main defenses are against the spoken word, so that interpretations have to be given in writing. Usually such children believe in the magic of words and realize that the analyst is saving them from the embarrassment and pain of the spoken word. For example, one little boy said quite definitely that he didn't mind what I talked to his parents about, so long as he didn't hear it. Sometimes "aids" become resistances, and it is more difficult to drop them.

Aids to interpretation may misfire or be misused. One patient responded to an interpretation put in terms of his friend's actions by saying to the therapist, "Don't bother me about other people's problems; I have enough of my own!"

ANNA FREUD   In some of these cases the aids to interpretation go along with the patient's defenses, in part at least. If the analyst goes straight against the defense, she arouses unpleasure—it does not matter whether this comes from the superego, from other people, or from fear of unconscious wishes. For example, if the analyst interprets too early a child's death wish against the mother or against the siblings, this arouses all sorts of unpleasures, such as superego strictures ("One doesn't kill people"), fear of losing the object, fear of the magical quality of one's wishes. By going slowly, by showing the child that she understands that there are children who fight with their mothers and who are very angry with them, or by showing in play that a particular doll really did want to kill the mother doll, the analyst comes a step nearer to the defended content. The child thinks, "Well, I'm not the only one, and it isn't as terrible as I had thought, and one can really talk about it without getting too criticized or too upset." To accept such feelings in oneself is a gradual process.

18

Significant Interpretations

Accounts of psychoanalytic interventions usually give special significance to particular interpretations; this is as true for reports of work with children as with adults. Certain special interpretations influence the analytic work at particular times in the analysis and are worth singling out for special attention. The questions of the significance of an interpretation and of the relationship between apparently significant interpretations and the remainder of the analytic work are important for all analysts.

Interpretations are considered significant when they bring about a shift in the patient's behavior or material. Such changes are not always manifested immediately after an interpretation is made for the first time. A period of working though is usually necessary, during which the interpretation may have to be repeated in different forms and different contexts. Often only after this period will the therapist see those changes in the child's material or behavior that demonstrate the significance of the interpretation. Certain patients show marked improvement in certain areas, and it is impossible for the therapist to identify and isolate the particularly significant interpretation that may have contributed to the change.

A "meaningful" interpretation was recorded in the case of eleven-and-one-half-year-old Frank O.:

In his fourth year of treatment, Frank's rivalry with his younger brother reappeared in the treatment material, this time in anal terms. While farting, Frank told the therapist about how much he hated his brother. He claimed not to be afraid of the "toilet noises" but admitted to a fear of being trapped

To Index: Record interpretations of particular importance, especially those that brought about a significant shift in the child's material or his behavior.

inside the toilet. This led to material about how his mother permitted the baby brother to soil and wet and even petted him, while she threw Frank's feces away with disgust. The therapist interpreted Frank's childhood wish to throw his brother down the lavatory, like feces, and she also verbalized the jealous fury at the mother he had experienced at that time. This evoked an explosion of destructive rage in the session—Frank smashed and threw the toys and furniture about, he threw plasticine at the therapist, and then he attacked her violently. Now the material became increasingly concerned with Frank's anger with his mother rather than anger at the brother. Thus, from talking about killing his brother and enacting sadistic executions, Frank began to play messily with water and plasticine, and he eventually splashed dirty water on the therapist's clothes. This was understood and interpreted to be a reenactment of episodes in which Frank tried to stop his mother from leaving him by dirtying her clothes when she got dressed up to go out. Frank's immediate response to this significant interpretation was agreement and relief. Subsequently the analytic material shifted from anal concerns to other areas, and concomitant changes in Frank's external functioning were noted. His teacher reported that his schoolwork advanced remarkably well within just a few days.

Coming from the fourth year of his treatment, the example of Frank's progress illustrates the fact that a great deal of analytic work usually precedes so-called significant interpretations. Earlier Frank's therapist had devoted much effort to work around the topic of his hostility to the brother and his fears of retaliation, especially as they related to his projection of anger and his guilty feelings about his mother's desertion when he was five years old. That material had emerged in relation to Frank's tormenting a kitten, an activity which was accompanied by much guilt and fear of retaliation. The therapist learned from the father that after Frank's brother had been born, the patient showed hardly any signs of jealousy of the baby or of anger toward his mother, but that for a while he severely tormented a kitten which his mother had "adopted" soon after coming home with the baby.

ANNA FREUD   If we analysts say that a significant interpretation is one which has brought about changes, we then have to examine how it works. We have to ask about the relations between interpretation and insight, for example, and we also have to take into account the patient's responses to interpretations.

The "significant" interpretations which brought such dramatic relief to Frank, with a subsequent impressive increase in his ability to learn, possibly did not result in the recovery of a memory as such, but rather in the recovery of affects and feelings relevant to earlier experiences. Perhaps the relief following the interpretation was a consequence of the fact that the more mature ego of the child was now better able to accept the hostile wishes, especially when they were seen by the patient to have links with the past.

Arthur H. began treatment at the age of twelve years four months; his material was indexed when he was thirteen years six months old:

In the eighteenth week of treatment, after a session in which he spoke of his discomfort in "performing" before others, he showed a return to modes of behavior seen earlier in treatment, including silence, looking at the therapist, coming near to convulsive giggling, and fiddling with a piece of plasticine. He was not responsive to the interpretation that he saw the therapist as an audience who expected him to perform, but continued with the plasticine play. After a considerable period of silence, the reconstruction was made that Arthur resembled a child sitting on a potty, who would not perform and thereby kept his mother waiting; that he was now "controlling" the therapist just as he must have done with his mother, making the therapist into the "waiting mother." Arthur reacted with great amusement and then spoke with a lively freedom of such battles now going on between his mother and three-and-one-half-year-old sister. He appeared to derive considerable vicarious satisfaction from the mother's helplessness in this sadomasochistic interaction. Attempts were then made to show Arthur how he felt criticized by the therapist for expressing his messy, anal-sadistic wishes, for example by his abandoning his messy painting once the therapist had commented on its character. Just as he feared in the past that mother would not stand for his messy behavior and would leave him if such expressions emerged, so he seemed to expect the same thing of the therapist. That these transference interpretations were most significant was suggested by his coming closer to free association in the following session and rarely reverting to such withholding behavior in subsequent treatment.

The example from Arthur's case may represent anal-sadistic regression in the transference, in which regressed material is produced and the interpretation given in terms of a revival of something that has taken place in the past. The interpretation Arthur received was effective in that the material came more freely in the next session, and this particular regression was rarely seen again in the analysis. The fact that Arthur's associations to the interpretation referred to the development of a parallel and contemporary situation with his younger sister and the mother can be taken as confirmatory material and can be regarded as part of the working-through process.

The particular reconstruction detailed in Arthur's example was based on the clues to the anal content, such as the fiddling with plasticine and the discomfort in performing before others. There had also been the change in Arthur's usual way of behaving in the sessions as well as in the controlling nature of his silence. All these were indications to the therapist that Arthur was behaving like a child on the potty. The eighteen months of analytic work that preceded this particular session had prepared the therapist for the situation in which the reconstruction was made. Effective interpretations are the culmination of processes which have been going on for a long time. Although on occasion it is possible to refer some change to a single step, therapists should not normally expect magical consequences of a "good" interpretation.

Certain patients show that a particular interpretation has had a special significance for them, continually returning to it or referring to it in one way or another. Hannah, a five-year-old girl who had not appeared to respond to any interpretations regarding her very evident angry feelings, was sung a song by her therapist with the refrain, "Little Hannah is cross." Hannah often returned to this song at appropriate moments later in treatment and asked the therapist to sing it to her again. The therapist's use of song as an aid to interpretation was successful because the song made the aggression more acceptable to the patient, probably because, by singing about it, the therapist conveyed the idea that she herself accepted it.

Interpretations have many different kinds of significance. Too precise a definition of significance would exclude many important interpretations. An interpretation may be "good" in that it has an effect on the subsequent analytic work. Interpretations may also be good because they include all the different aspects of a conflict and are followed by working through over a period of time and over a broad area. Other interpretations may be felt to be good by the therapist because they pull things together in the therapist's mind, even though they are not particularly effective when conveyed to the patient.

Significant interpretations do not just happen. They are preceded by other analytic work, work which includes prior interpretations and other interventions by the therapist. Moreover, an interpretation may bring about a progressive shift in the child's development and behavior because it reduces an anxiety which previously prevented such a shift. A child may have regressed in the face of anxiety brought about, for example, by conflict, and his behavior may be dominated by the regressively revived fantasies, impulses, and modes of functioning. The interpretation of the child's anxiety, from which he had retreated, might permit him to move forward again, and the content of the regression-dominated behavior need not be included in the "significant" interpretation.

19

Selection and Timing

The analyst is always faced with problems of selecting relevant and important aspects of the material in order to direct his interpretations toward the most significant and immediate areas. Timing of interpretations is also crucial. Although it is not possible to lay down rules for interpretation, it is possible to enumerate certain guiding principles. The selection and timing of interpretations is an extremely important subject, cutting across many fundamental issues in psychoanalytic technique.

The patient herself may indicate that material selected for interpretation is inappropriate or that it is inappropriately timed, as did Susan S., the six-and-one-half-year-old who was treated from the age of three years one month because of emotional disturbances associated with constitutional sexual precocity:

Following a period during which Susan began to make strides in her ego achievements, it became clear that she resisted interpretations because she experienced them as seductions. Thus, for example, when the therapist interpreted her fear that she had damaged herself through masturbation, Susan said that the therapist's talking made her too hot and she wished she had a zipper to put on the therapist's mouth. At this point, the therapist decided to avoid further reference to this particular content, which was sexually exciting to the child, and decided instead to lend support to the developmental moves which were taking place. For example, Susan once brought material which showed her penis envy of her brother and father by talking

To Index: Note instances when the selection of material for interpretation and the timing of interpretations have special importance for the subsequent development of the treatment process. Note both appropriate and inappropriate timing, as well as factors affecting the choice of and emphasis on material. State the reasons for adopting a particular technique (e.g. the need to deal first with a reality situation rather than the patient's fantasies).

about the former's magic toy and the latter's big garden hose. Susan then played at sitting at a desk and writing, at which point the therapist took up Susan's wish to find ways to identify with males through male activities.

The discomfort Susan expressed when it was brought up led the therapist to avoid an overtly sexual topic and the associated guilt and to turn instead to the little girl's wish to be a boy and to her efforts to augment her self-esteem by identifying with a man's activities. Her reason for doing this was in order to avoid overexciting the child, in the knowledge that the sexualization of all her experiences was a significant problem for her and that her recent ego achievements indicated some increase in her capacity to cope with this particular difficulty. Because Susan's resistance to interpretations may have been evoked by the therapist's reference to Susan's masturbation, it might have been possible for the therapist to circumvent the resistances or the excitement by taking up the embarrassment or guilt feelings related to masturbation. For Susan, sexual excitement was an all-pervasive phenomenon, with openly displayed masturbation. Therefore it should not be regarded as defensive, as sexual excitement so often is in anxiety-laden situations.

The degree of sexualization shown by Susan is unusual for her age group. In the process of establishing latency it is more common that a child distances himself from direct sexual expressions by use of displacements, proxies, and symbolic material. Therefore it is more usual in child analysis for the therapist to approach sexual content beginning with surface or more distant material and only gradually working toward the underlying sexual fantasies and wishes. But in the experience of some therapists the opposite holds: a direct discussion of sexual material is often quite acceptable to the preschool child or even the latency child. Much must depend on the degree of embarrassment which the child has about sexual material, about his own masturbation and associated fantasies, about his wishes to be of the opposite sex. Often young children are quite ready to discuss subjects which are sensitive for older children and adults.

In the case of Frank O. an entirely different kind of reality factor influenced the selection and timing of interpretations. The indexing was done when Frank was aged eight years eight months, after one year of treatment:

Because it was recognized almost as soon as he began treatment that Frank was currently deprived of adequate maternal care and had from the beginning turned to his therapist to satisfy this need, the treatment remained primarily concerned with current reality problems. There were many indications of earlier difficulties given in symbolic play, difficulties over death wishes toward siblings and oedipal material. These were on the whole understood by the therapist but not interpreted at the time. Until arrangements could be made for a suitable housekeeper to be engaged, it was not felt by the therapist to be appropriate for him to take up Frank's present conflicts in terms of his experience of his mother's desertion when he was five years old.

Some patients, like Frank, are experiencing current, overwhelmingly distressing reality which must be taken into account by the therapist in choosing what to interpret and when.

ANNA FREUD A situation such as Frank's is certainly not the best time either to reach the problems of the past or in fact to reach anything unrelated to the present stress or deprivation. In most instances like this, the analyst has to wait until the current problems subside before being able to take up other material effectively. It is the same in the analysis of adults. This is because the affect of the patient is wholly engaged in the present and not, as is often said, because the preoccupation with the present stress serves as a resistance to analysis.

The therapist might have less difficulty in selecting the time and area of interpretation if she constantly keeps in mind and follows the patient's preconscious preoccupations. If the preoccupation is related to a current situation with which the patient is having to cope, then the interventions of the therapist should be directed toward the patient's essential concerns. For a child who has just lost a parent through death, the initial reaction is of course discussed in the analysis. But as time goes by, the patient's reactions may change, and the therapist may see the development, for example, of guilt feelings owing to the patient's belief that his own wishes had brought about the death. Interpretation of such guilt feelings can be of great value in helping the patient to cope with the internal problems stimulated by the real change in the external circumstances. This is not necessarily identical with the process of analyzing what is going on in the person in terms of the patient's past. Indeed the past need not be relevant to what should be interpreted in relation to the patient's real, current problems. In addition to extreme and dramatic events such as the death of a parent, there are more chronic situations, such as the real deprivation experienced by Frank. Both extreme and chronic circumstances may necessitate postponement of analytic work proper until the child's reality needs are dealt with. There are also children who are exposed to violent parental quarrels at home, events that may significantly influence material they bring to subsequent sessions. The therapist should always be alert for such "intrusions" from the outside into the normal psychological unfolding of the analytic process.

It is possible that external influences may play a greater part in child analysis than in adult analysis. A child's turning away from the current analytic work should not automatically be understood as resistance to analysis. The therapist need not be totally silent about such a change, nor should she commiserate with the child only in case of major upsets such as a death. However, if the therapist follows the path of the child's preoccupations, it is unlikely that the work will remain focused exclusively on external factors. Ideally, the therapist follows the child's current internal adaptations and defenses as they evolve in coping with the external events and crises. This makes it possible for the therapist to make the appropriate interventions.

ANNA FREUD   This leaves open the question of where the child's emotions are at that moment. Are they available for the analytic work or are they wholly concerned with questions like, "Can I make mother come back, can I bring mother and father together again?" It is very much like trying to talk with someone in an acute state of pain when his mind is not really open to anything else.

The cases of Susan and Frank have concerned more the influence of external factors than issues of selection and timing per se. Although in Frank's case the provision of an adequate care-taking person was necessary before the patient could avail himself of analysis, other children may bring material early in the analysis through play much like Frank's without needing attention to external factors in their lives. Given symbolic material by a child with less immediate needs than Frank's, the therapist is confronted with considerations of selection and timing relatively uninfluenced by external events. It is very necessary to differentiate between the problem of phrasing an interpretation so that the unconscious and repressed material can be made conscious and acceptable to the patient, on the one hand, and the problem of choosing the right time to give the interpretation to the patient, on the other. Whereas the therapist may understand the meaning of what is going on in the patient, he may not be ready to accept this information because he has not yet been adequately prepared for it, or because it is not fully alive in him, although its presence is clearly shown in a variety of derivatives. Some patients flood the therapist with so much material that the therapist does not have the problem of selection and timing but rather a problem of understanding the mass of material presented to him.

Particular problems of the timing and selection of interpretations exist at the beginning of treatment, when the therapist does not yet have the benefit of the past analytic work with the patient as a guide. A typical situation of this sort arises when the child brings abundant material when treatment starts, but no distinct theme. The therapist must discern what should be taken up, as the therapist of Douglas O. had to. Douglas was fifteen years three months at the beginning of treatment and sixteen years seven months old when the indexing was done:

In the first weeks of treatment Douglas brought in a great deal of material through conscious worries, fantasies, and discussions of his obsessional symptoms and rituals. His accompanying affects were extreme distress and anxiety. The main themes Douglas presented were concerned with his present homosexual impulses and wishes, together with strong defenses against them, and his sadistic heterosexual fantasies and intense aggressive impulses, with the defenses against these. The problem of where to start in the face of such a mass of material as well as of Douglas's intense anxiety was urgent and difficult. There were no obvious links between his distress and the material he brought. It was finally decided to start with the aggressive murderous impulses because the patient seemed to put more emphasis on these. The other impulses, such as the homosexual ones, were more defended against and less accessible, probably because they were reinforced and became more threatening when Douglas found himself alone with a male therapist.

The therapist had thought at first that Douglas was simply showing an intense anxiety about beginning treatment and so attempted to address the anxiety first. As in many similar cases, the patient defended against his anxiety by "flooding" the hour with material, which made the interpretation ineffectual. It was because another approach was needed that the therapist, following the patient's material, chose the most accessible point in terms of what was relatively less defended against: Douglas's hostile and murderous impulses. In those cases in which hostile and aggressive material is a defense against anxiety connected with starting treatment, however, only the interpretation of the anxiety can really be effective.

A younger child, Calvin S., who began treatment at the age of four years five months and whose case was indexed when he was aged six years two months, required a very cautious approach to interpretation:

Calvin came to treatment because of an increasing difficulty at school, including a learning problem and a reluctance to go to school. By the third month of treatment Calvin was becoming reluctant to come to treatment. This was a consequence of the therapist's focusing on Calvin's defensive use of fantasy play. For example, Calvin insisted that the therapist should stick closely to roles assigned to him and should play without talking—that is, without interpreting links between the play and worrying reality events outside treatment. The therapist chose to take up Calvin's wish for help and commented on the two parts of Calvin that were in conflict—the part that did not want treatment and the part that wanted help. Finally, the therapist said that Calvin's talking about his worries in treatment reminded Calvin of worries outside the clinic. This made Calvin not want to come to treatment. Calvin listened attentively and said he would be angry if the therapist did not help him to gather up the toys. The therapist complied and pointed out that if Calvin were to be angry with him, he would feel naughty because of that, and then the therapist would become a frightening person to him. After this Calvin imagined a ghost and he enlisted the therapist's help in killing it. This was one of the first times he used the therapist as a "helper" in his fantasy play.

Calvin resisted interpretations which connected his play with his worries. The therapist was confronted with the choice of taking up and interpreting this resistance, or of first taking up another element. He chose to focus on an aspect of the treatment alliance which could then be linked with the resistance by verbalizing the child's conflict for him. If the therapist were to have taken up the content directly, he might have done so by saying something like, "You want to stop me from talking because you feel that I am attacking you." The therapist most likely thought that the latter approach would heighten the resistance and perhaps lead to phobic reaction in which the treatment or the therapist would become the feared object. In fact the therapist had been alerted to this possibility because of the reason for Calvin's referral, his incipient school phobia.

In general with any patient it is more advantageous to make interpretations step by step, as was done with Calvin, rather than by undercutting defenses and resistances by a direct interpretation of content. Certainly, many different paths can be taken in reaching an interpretation. The therapist may proceed by steps along any one of many different paths and yet reach the same ultimate goal. There is no "correct" path, although some ways of proceeding are smoother or more direct than others.

20

Working Through

Working through is as much a task of therapy as is interpretation itself. It reflects both the elaboration and the extension of the relevant interpretation in different contexts and directions. The patient's behavior and mental life gradually take in and integrate new knowledge and patterns of behavior as the process of working through proceeds.

There are at least two different ways of looking at the process of working through. According to one, the "work" involved is the tracing of all the various manifestations of a particular conflict, or of some particular solution to a conflict, in many areas. In the other view, the same situation appears repeatedly in the analysis and is interpreted again in more or less the same way, perhaps with slight variations, resulting in a progressive withdrawal of some of the patient's investment in a particular pattern of mental activity or behavior.

The success of the process of working through depends on the therapist's awareness that the interpretation itself is not magic. A great deal of work has to be done in preparation for the interpretation, and working through is a consolidation of this work, whether in the session or outside it.

ANNA FREUD Working through can be seen as the elaboration and
the extension of the interpretation in different contexts. To a
greater extent with children than with adults, more of what the

To Index: Note instances of working through. Give examples of the relevant
interpretations, and if possible note whether the working through occurred inside
or outside the treatment hour.

182

therapist has interpreted tends to slip away and to reappear in a new form, when it has to be interpreted again. It is really the constant reiteration of the interpretation that serves the working-through process, especially with the child. In my very first book on child analysis, I gave a striking example of this in regard to a little girl who is now a grandmother. She had great penis envy, which I interpreted busily and repeatedly; she understood it and accepted it. She had an elder brother whom she envied very much. The patient was a very masculine little girl at the time—but she took the problem of her penis envy seriously. She came one day and said that now she really understood it, and that there was just no sense in always envying boys. After all, what boys had was not so important. What she would really like to be was an elephant, because they had such a wonderful trunk. So there was the whole problem once again, and it made me very thoughtful at the time. The problem just took on another disguise. This is characteristic of what occurs in all analyses, but is perhaps more frequently met in children. I had an adult patient who used me in the transference for masochistic purposes. For example, he came ten or fifteen minutes early for an early morning hour, and if I was not there at the time, he acted as if I were fifteen minutes late; he had an elaborate grievance about this. In his analysis I used the example about the elephant to show him how he invented his grievances and built them up and what he got from them. He understood this very well. The next day he complained in much the usual way about the previous day's interpretation, that I accused him of manufacturing grievances, whereas everybody manufactures grievances. Without knowing it, he had produced exactly the same grievance with another rationalization.

Working through seems to be as much a task for the therapist as for the patient. In fact, a technical aspect of the therapist's work is to be aware of the working through needed in regard to further extensions of previously interpreted material.

ANNA FREUD   Long ago I reported the case of a little boy with severe anxiety symptoms. I had scarcely analyzed the anxiety in one form when it appeared in another. Finally he said, "Do you think it is really sensible that you chase it around like that?" A distinction must be made between tracing material that appears in different contexts and tracing the appearance of the same difficulty repeatedly but in lesser and lesser degree. Analysts must face the question of when to be satisfied that sufficient working through has taken place.

It might be said that sufficient working through has taken place when the child has moved to the next level of development and established himself there. The process of working through in child analysis is simultaneous with ordinary structural development in the psychological sphere. This is not quite the same as what is found in adult analysis, where working through is one of the causes of structural change which might not occur without it. In adult analysis working through could be regarded as a way of reinforcing structural change brought about through appropriate interpretation. With children, change occurs all the time, and the process of working through interacts with such normal change.

Psychoanalytic work with children has shown that working through is not limited to the therapeutic session. Reinforcement and "practice" occur outside the therapy hour, and the child often reports how he has applied bits of insight which might have been gained during the therapy, possibly because the main objects of the child during his analysis are still the parents. The therapist can provide insight and understanding which will immediately affect the child's relations to his parents or other significant figures.

A clinical example of working through comes from the case of Greta F., indexed when she was four years eight months old, two years after treatment began:

Greta could use play for the purpose of mastering anxiety arising either from the analytic work or from other sources. For example, she would enact in play at home something which was current in the analysis and verbalized there. This seemed to serve integration and working through. At the age of three years three months, Greta's fear of her mother's leaving her became the focus of the analytic work. At one point she recalled that her mother had left her in a pram with a neighbor. Following this, she introduced a game with her dolls at home in which she played that her mother was busy while Greta napped. It appeared that this was Greta's way of working through her anxiety, and subsequently she was able to take naps without her mother's physical presence.

The memory Greta confronted during the course of treatment, involving the fear of her mother leaving her, was a very painful one. Although the case shows the way in which the patient coped with the internal problems aroused by the memory, it does not include the actual interpretations given to the patient. Certainly the memory was not all that was involved; Greta was also confronted with her anxiety that her mother would desert her. She felt that such a desertion was imminent. The analyst's task was to present the fact that her mother was not about to desert her, but that the child was fearful of it because she had experienced it that way earlier.

Greta was able to work through this material in doll play at home rather than in the session, probably because for her, as for many young children, the mother of the present also served as the transference object for the mother of the past. Greta's play at home could be considered to be a resistance in the form of the acting out of material which properly belonged in the session, but this view is probably more appropriate for adults and perhaps older children in analysis. The concept of working through is linked to the concept of resistance in the sense that there are constant efforts made by the patient to avoid painful feelings. Working through is often pitted directly against resistance.

ANNA FREUD   There are dangers in making assumptions about children in analysis which parallel assumptions frequently made about adult treatment. For example, in Greta's case the assumption would be that if she remembered at the age of three that she had been left in a pram at the age of one, this would free her from anxiety. It is not very likely that a child at three remembers being left in the pram at the age of one year. It is more probable that the experience of being left and of finding herself suddenly without the mother had a traumatic effect on the child. This created a fear of similar situations and a marked lack of confidence in the mother's reliability. What treatment deals with currently is this distrust, which is a developmental consequence of the traumatic situation. The discovery of the memory of being left in the pram is not what brings about the therapeutic change; instead, change is brought about by the gradual confrontation of the patient with the mother as she really is, as distinct from the child's fantasy image of the mother. Some analysts offer such interpretations to a child in treatment as, "You were hungry when you were six months old and your feeds came too slowly." Their rationale for this approach is that it is curative, but the interpretation, or the recovery of the memory, does not have this effect. The belief of analysts that the interpretation of early trauma has a relatively immediate curative effect is based on their transferring to such interpretation their experience of the fact that the interpretation of unconscious internalized conflict often quickly assists the therapeutic process.

Whereas with some adult patients the recovery of a childhood traumatic experience, either spontaneously or as a consequence of interpretation, is often accompanied by relief and possibly permanent change in the patient, this does not apply to young children. Early traumas can be interpreted to young children, but even if the memory is recovered, there is nothing equivalent to the abreaction which may occur in adult patients. In child analysis the interpretation is of value only if it increases the child's understanding of what is currently happening. There is a crucial difference between analyzing neurotic conflicts and tracing anxieties which are consequent on the child's infantile perception of the world. In young children an earlier distortion of perception due to the immaturity of the child's perceptual and cognitive apparatus may lead to anxiety or to some other disturbance; the analytic task is to correct the faulty reality which had been registered earlier. This task is very different from interpreting an internal or internalized conflict and is also relevant to the subject of working through.

21

Restrictions

In this area of child analysis, as in many others, technical difficulties arise when the model of treatment technique for adults is applied indiscriminately, without modification, for the treatment of children. In the adult treatment situation the adult has complete freedom of verbal expression, which is usually sufficient for the analytic process to proceed satisfactorily. Because the child does not have the same capacity to express everything verbally, other modes of expression are allowed and in fact neccessary. By its very nature, however, the child analytic treatment situation imposes restrictions on the child in that it cannot offer complete freedom of expression. It is often necessary for the therapist to discourage or even prohibit certain forms of behavior in the child. Occasionally even physical restraints have to be imposed in order to permit the analytic work to proceed. With children, interpretation of the behavior is often insufficient to bring about its modification.

Certain children accept the limitations of the analytic setting from the beginning but at certain periods of the analysis test the limits or transgress them. Other patients rebel from the start against what they feel to be the restrictions of the analytic setting.

ANNA FREUD The analyst never says to an adult patient at the beginning of analysis, "This is a place where you can do whatever you want," or "This is a place of complete freedom." Some child

---

To Index: Record any restriction, prohibition, or restraint explicitly imposed on the child in the analytic setting if it is a significant or unusual feature of the treatment. Note the circumstances leading to the restriction, its repercussions, and its meaning for the child.

analysts imply this to the patients, however. With the adult, the analyst lays down clearly what the restrictions are, as they relate to time, to talking instead of acting, and so on. There is a whole set of rules, with various reasons for them. For example, the primary purpose for the rule requiring the adult patient to lie on the couch is to serve verbal expression, which also may facilitate regression. With children, expression cannot be limited to verbalization alone, and therefore analysts provide toys and the playroom. Here the problem in regard to restrictions begins.

Some children may experience the analytic setting as such as a restriction, as when the child is restricted to the treatment room or to the toys available there. Indeed, the very commitment by the parents to bring or send the child to analysis imposes a restriction on the child's spontaneous activity. This is different from the situation in adult analysis where, if the patient does not come, he knows that it is his own loss, and he has to pay for his missed session. The child is under pressure from the parents to come even if he does not want to, and if he misses a session, it is the parents who have to pay and who suffer. On the whole, children accept the analytic setting at the outset, whether they perceive it in terms of restrictions, conditions, or promises. The difference between the treatment of adults and children in this regard is that the transgressions of and protests against the analytic conditions are verbalized more often by the adult but enacted more frequently by the child. In addition, the child patient's tendency to enact is facilitated by the regression and disinhibition which may occur during analysis. Such enactments cannot always be adequately interpreted and may interfere with the progress of the analytic work unless the therapist also puts restrictions on the child's behavior.

Although the tendency of the child to regress during analysis may necessitate restrictions, a certain amount of regression is desirable for the progress of the analysis. A delicate balance must be maintained by the therapist in order to foster the progressive development of the child and, at the same time, to be able to work with material which has been produced by the regressive revival of the past. Accordingly, it may be unproductive to provide materials, such as water and sand, which encourage regression in the treatment room;

instead, materials such as paint and modeling clay may be preferable, because although they to some extent allow regression, they also provide a suitable means of expression for the child. Techniques which encourage or facilitate regression of the sort that involves nonverbal modes of expression are to be avoided.

Paul Q. was three years four months old at the beginning of treatment and four years six months at the time of indexing:

In the first six weeks of treatment Paul was frequently very aggressive and attacking toward the therapist, trying to bite, kick, and scratch her, as well as throwing toys at her. The therapist physically restrained Paul while verbalizing Paul's anger, in order to control his outbursts and to allow him to feel supported by her and less overwhelmed by his anger. When released, he would run out of the room, returning to yell rather than physically to attack. During this period of the analysis, the therapist removed the heavier toys, which otherwise were used as missiles. At a later stage in the treatment, Paul tried to run out of the treatment room and the clinic into the street whenever he was overwhelmed by panic. At these times the therapist picked up the patient and carried him indoors to safety, feeling that physically holding and protecting him was necessary at this point.

The therapist always has to be ready to impose restrictions on the child, for good reason: it is done to protect the child, the therapist, and the environment. By this protection it is hoped to keep the child safe, to prevent him from feeling too anxious and guilty about his behavior, and to facilitate the continuation of the analysis. Ultimately these aims are best accomplished by encouraging the child to bring material as far as possible verbally or through fantasy play, in this way enabling him to accept his unconscious wishes rather than to act them out. Along with this development in the child goes the child's ability to make progressively better distinctions between the enactment of a wish and the wish itself.

ANNA FREUD   Early in the history of child analysis it was thought that acting out, and especially the release of aggression, was in itself therapeutic. Nowadays one occasionally still hears this expressed in the idea that the child must be given a lot of leeway in his behavior, because what is unconscious will reveal itself better in "free expression." This is not so. On the contrary, the analytic material is obscured and changed if the analyst permits a massive regression in this way.

Andy V., who was two years six months when analysis began, was three years two months old when this example was indexed:

Andy had to be restrained on several occasions, particularly when he pulled at the towel bar, which he finally managed to pull away from the wall, and the not well-fixed washbasin, and also when, at the climax of his washing games, he splashed water all over the place. Verbal comment by the therapist was usually along the lines that the therapist would not allow Andy to hurt him or to cause too much damage. Restraint varied from lifting him bodily away from the object he was attacking to pulling out the plug and tightening the taps. Responses were invariably fury at the therapist and sometimes retaliatory physical attack.

In Andy's example the age of the child is relevant, because it is age-appropriate for such a young child to rely on the adult for control. As the therapist was restraining Andy, he told him why he did so. In some cases the therapist may be able to interpret the unconscious reasons for the child's behavior. Anna Freud has emphasized that in adult analysis there are no limits to free association, whereas in child analysis there are limits to action. An important question for child therapists is just where to set the limits on action. Restrictions imposed in the treatment situation are different from ordinary restrictions at home or school because they are accompanied by the therapist's verbalizations and, if possible, interpretations. Outside treatment, such restrictions are more often accompanied by moralizing or by chastising the child. A clear differentiation should be made between restrictions that become necessary during the course of the analysis and the imposition of so-called discipline on the child.

Some therapists believe that a problem cannot be adequately analyzed if any restrictions at all are imposed on the child's behavior. They believe that, by resorting to restrictions, they make themselves into the kind of superego figure they do not want to be. But different children require different limits, and therapists vary in what they can tolerate comfortably. There are many therapists who are quite reluctant to do analysis while forcibly restraining a child, although, as Anna Freud has pointed out, this too depends on the child's age and pathology. Most child therapists have had the experience of making effective interpretations while physically restraining the child.

It is likely that children's sexual strivings are more readily deflected than are aggressive urges by restrictions or limitations imposed during treatment. Something of a social sense of shame about sex probably enters into the treatment situation, whereas shame may not apply in the same way to aggressive impulses. Children seem to feel less embarrassed about allowing themselves to behave aggressively than about sexual behavior of one sort or another.

Ilse T. was another patient who displayed aggression during analytic sessions. Four years eleven months old when she began treatment, Ilse was aged six years six months when the material was indexed:

In Ilse's treatment there were occasions when her provocations and attacks on the therapist, such as attempts to cut her clothes or smear her with plasticine, had to be physically restrained. She sometimes reacted to this restraint with giggles. Her need to make the therapist cross and her pleasure from it was interpreted in terms of the teasing love relationship she had with her mother.

Ilse's therapist actually restrained her physically, at the same time appropriately interpreting her enactment in the transference, thus encouraging verbal expression.

There are various reasons why a child might behave differently in the treatment situation from the way he does at home or school. Besides displaying aggressive behavior in sessions, children sometimes express strong curiosity or become sexually excited in the session. They may also test the limits in order to assess the therapist's tolerance for and acceptance of them. It may be necessary for the therapist to say rather early in the analysis, in response to a piece of provocative behavior, "I know you are only doing that to try me out, so tell me what you want to do next." Such a statement can serve as an interpretation, but it also invites the child to express things on a verbal level. The situation becomes difficult if the therapist uses it to try to prove that he does not get angry like the mother, because the child can always find some action which eventually has to be stopped. He needs only to try to jump out of the window. The therapist should aim for early interpretation of the activity rather than complete permissiveness. With some children of the testing sort one might have to say, "I know you are trying me out, but I can tell you that I will just have to stop you like Mommy does." Or, alternatively, "How far do you want me to let you go? We both know I will have to stop you at some time." These are all examples of using an analytic technique while still imposing a restriction of action.

22

Physical Contact and Gratification

The differences in technique between child and adult analysis concerning physical contact and gratification are determined not by any difference of analytic principle but rather by the differences which exist between the child and the adult. Experiences of physical contact or gratification are not themselves technical measures or deliberate acts.

In child analysis there are occasions when the therapist might find it necessary to become directly involved in the actual satisfaction of the wishes and needs of the patient. For example, with a young child a situation may arise which requires the therapist to take the child to the toilet or to help him put his clothes on. With older children, technical problems may focus on whether to provide food or drink or to permit toys to be taken home.

It would be quite unnatural to refuse assistance to a child who needs it, to refuse help with undoing a button or with tying shoelaces when the child cannot do the task for himself. In fact, not giving such needed help might very well keep the therapist distant from aspects of the child's inner life. It is one thing, however, to tie the shoelaces of a three-year-old and quite another for a nine-year-old. The therapist has to keep in mind the age-appropriateness of the child's requests for help and his general level of ego functioning, including his ability to tolerate frustration and anxiety.

A seven-year-old girl came to the first session of her analysis wearing a light summer dress, suitable for the weather at the time.

To Index: Describe incidents of physical involvement with patients or the gratification of physical needs. Explain the rationale for decisions in this area and the effect they have on the analytic work.

On entering the basement treatment room, she shivered and said she was cold. The therapist, who was aware that this room was unusually cold and had dressed accordingly, acknowledged that it was indeed cold and inquired if the patient had brought a sweater. Because she had not and because she continued shivering, the therapist offered the child his jacket, which was accepted gratefully. This therapist met a patient's realistic need in an appropriate way. It can be argued that it may have been sexually stimulating for a seven-year-old girl to wear the male therapist's jacket or that, since this was a first session, this is not a typical example of meeting a patient's realistic need in an appropriate way. The patient did not know beforehand, as the therapist did, that this room was cold. The therapist would most likely respond differently in subsequent sessions if such a situation were to recur. The fact that this was the first session may have influenced the therapist for other reasons as well, in particular because of his wish to foster a treatment alliance.

As in many situations, this child's gratification was a "normal" by-product of the way the therapist dealt with her at the time. The therapist's action may have had other incidental implications, just as any piece of behavior on the part of the therapist may have further implications for the child. There are many situations in which the child seems actively to seek physical contact in order to obtain gratification from this. These situations can range from cuddling up to the therapist or wanting to sit on the therapist's lap, to trying on the therapist's jewelry or aggressively pulling off the therapist's shoes. The technical problem is how to permit the child optimal expression of his unconscious wishes and fantasies without his experiencing overexcitement or rejection. Some attempts to restrict the more energetic behavior that children often display in analysis may involve physical contact, which may then, incidentally, be gratifying to the patient.

One child may come to the hour feeling hungry and ask for a cookie or a drink; another may simply demand food constantly without any particular immediate cause. Some children ask the therapist for candy; some bring their own. There are children who feed their therapists, like the little girl who would not talk until the therapist ate the candy the patient brought with her. Such material may be meaningful beyond simple direct gratification, as in the case of the frightened child who defensively stuffs himself with food. The difference between giving sweets and providing play material may be considered an arbitrary one, because ultimately the question is whether or not the therapist should provide something, rather than a question of exactly what is provided. In a clinic there may be a somewhat artificial division between the receptionist in the waiting room, who may appropriately provide juice and cookies to the child who comes to treatment after school, and the therapists, who do not. This division of function between the receptionist and the therapist may be a critical one from the point of view of the analysis.

In child analysis the therapist cannot help but be a provider in many ways. For some children, the therapist's role as a provider of some sort is crucial to the progress of the analytic work.

ANNA FREUD   The taboo on gratifying a request for sweets in the analytic hour is unjust, for sweets are singled out from all the other things that are given. Sweets may be extremely important to one child, whereas the toy or kit or whatever it is that a child is in love with may be equally important to another. Children so often complain to their therapist, "You didn't get me the toy I wanted," or express satisfaction by saying, "You thought of it and you gave it to me." It is the demanding, the giving, and the receiving which are much more important than what is demanded, given, or received.

Showing the child that he is "thought of" applies equally to Christmas or birthday presents. At times, particularly with very young children, the giving of such presents may be a necessary and appropriate part of the relationship.

The problem of a child's wish to take toys home arose in the case of Jerry N., who was four years four months when treatment began and six years four months when the example was indexed:

During the early stages of Jerry's analysis, when he was very upset at weekends and afraid that he would not be able to return on Monday, he was allowed to take a toy home with him over the weekend.

Often at the beginning of treatment the therapist comes to an agreement with the child about toys, for instance that the toys are for the child's exclusive use in the treatment room and will be safely kept for him there. Individual lockers may be provided for each child, with keys kept by the therapists. Rules have to be flexible, and in certain instances, as in the example of Jerry, exceptions should be made. Very often a therapist is confronted with a child's demands to take things home at one stage or another. The meanings behind such demands vary enormously, and the therapist develops a greater understanding of the meaning of a particular child's demands as his knowledge of the child increases. On the basis of the increased knowledge he can gratify or refuse such demands.

In one of Anna Freud's earliest cases, a boy of five frequently begged to take a toy home. Anna Freud invariably found that these toys were dropped in the anteroom. The child did not wish to take the toy home as a way of dealing with the separation; rather, it was the battle with his therapist which was uppermost in his mind. The toy was quite irrelevant in this case, Anna Freud knew, but by permitting the child to take the toy and then seeing what he did with it, she could understand what it was used for.

Paul Q.'s case provides more information about the nature of a child's fears manifested by the wish to take toys home. Paul began treatment at the age of three years four months and was indexed when he was four years six months of age:

On certain occasions Paul insisted on being allowed to take his toy snake, his pieces of wood, his paintbox, and his airplane out of the treatment room because he feared that a burglar might come and steal them. The analysis revealed that these articles represented things he would like to steal from rivals, and that the fear of the burglar was a consequence of his projected aggressive wish. When interpretation of the fear was not sufficient to enable him to leave these toys behind without panic, the therapist permitted him to take them home.

The therapist went along with Paul's fear because it was not amenable to interpretation. What this example does not make clear is the fact that it often takes considerable time to analyze such fears. In such a situation a therapist is confronted with the technical problem of what to do in the meantime, especially when the child's defenses against his anxiety include wishes to take toys home. Simply saying no may cause the child to experience the therapist as dangerous, creating more resistance. Or the child may get very angry with the therapist, to the detriment of the analysis at that particular point.

Fulfilling the child's wish may be necessary as a temporary expedient to be used by the therapist in order to enable the relevant material to be analyzed later.

Occasionally a child insists on doing homework in the analytic hour. If the therapist helps him with the work during the session, it may lessen the child's anxiety at school. In some cases, however, doing so only postpones the outbreak of a severe anxiety attack in the session. This raises a dilemma. On the one hand, if the therapist persists in giving in to the patient's defenses against anxiety, he may remain unaware of the magnitude of the hidden anxiety in the patient. On the other hand, if he refuses from the beginning to allow the patient to do his homework in the hour, the child might not be able to cooperate with the analytic work because of his general level of anxiety. At the beginning, the therapist might think that doing the homework is merely a resistance and an effort to block the analytic process, whereas it might be that the demand for help is to ward off an immense anxiety having to do with the school situation.

Permitting a child to take materials home or helping him to do homework in the session are not necessarily or simply gratifications. The requests and permissions can have a variety of meanings for the child. A skilled therapist tries to be in the position of enabling the child to contain his anxieties while continuing the analysis of them.

The case of Charles Z. is a more complicated one than the cases presented thus far and illustrates a somewhat older child's demands. Charles began treatment when eleven years four months old, and the indexing was done when he was fourteen years one month old:

For a long time in his analysis, Charles made many demands to take things home, declaring that he needed paper and pencils for work at home. His reactions to frustration in general were so intense that the therapist sometimes felt it advisable partially to satisfy a demand so as to forestall extreme despair. However, the therapist consistently interpreted transference aspects in which Charles experienced the therapist as being like his mother, whom he felt withheld what was due to him. Later in treatment Charles's demands were tempered so that they took the form of requests by Charles to borrow various desired objects, promising to return them. When he did return these things, he always made comments aimed at making the therapist feel greedy for taking such trivial things back from him.

Charles was making demands for gratification which were part of the transference. A therapist must determine just how much frustration to allow a child to experience. After all, there are many children who demonstrate their greed as well as their anxieties by their demandingness. It may be extremely difficult for the therapist to estimate how much frustration the child can tolerate and still participate in the analytic work. Sometimes a compromise understanding may be reached with the child that material will be rationed. He may be given, for example, one model kit per month or four pieces of drawing paper per session. The important thing is always the continuation of the analytic work, and denying the child's requests may at times lead to an interference with the work; therefore, temporary compromises may have to be reached. There are some therapists who seem very ready to allow the child certain gratifications because they are afraid of losing the case. Or a therapist may allow gratifications because she fears the transference may otherwise be adversely affected (if she becomes "a bad lady who says no,") evoking an unanalyzable resistance. In general, therapists who express fear of adversely affecting the transference really mean that they are afraid of disturbing the positive transference, and their fears of refusing certain gratifications may be rationalizations they use in order to avoid the child's hostile feelings. This is a countertransference problem.

ANNA FREUD   In doing analysis, the analyst has to act as one does when one wants to land a fish, by pulling it in only when one has caught it. If the analyst sticks too inflexibly to a rule, he may not get hold of the material. The analyst alternates between complying with the patient's wish and complying with the analytic rule, sometimes giving in, sometimes interpreting beforehand, sometimes only afterward. The main thing is to get hold of the material, but one important rule is not to collude with the patient. For example, a patient's phobic mechanism cannot be analyzed if the analyst colludes with it. However, I doubt that a child can be analyzed by constantly refusing all his demands. In fact, I do not see how anyone can carry through a child analysis without providing something concrete that a child wants, at one point or another in the analysis. The situation can be looked at this way: a child needs inducements, fulfillments, or satisfactions (others may call them bribes)—whereas the adult has other inducements—to carry on the analytic work.

Rather than establishing rules per se, the therapist can set forth guidelines or limits for the particular child as part of the frame of reference for the analytic setting as treatment gets under way. Thus the therapist may let a child make a mess, but only to a certain degree. The therapist may gratify a child, but again only give a certain amount. Guidelines as to what is appropriate and what is inappropriate can be gained by considering the patient's age and disturbance. We also have to take into account the therapist's tolerance. On the whole, water and sand should not be provided, but sometimes exceptions can be made. Usually such material is not given to the child because of the regressive pull of such play material and other reasons, but they should not be absolutely barred, even though their provision may create practical problems for the therapist.

23

Modifications of Technique

With very young children and with adolescents, with physically handicapped children (blind or deaf, for example), and with delinquent and borderline patients, the therapist must often introduce variations in technique. This may also be necessary in the treatment of particular disturbances, such as those in which anxiety manifests itself in an inability to stay in the treatment room, to speak with the therapist, or to permit the therapist to speak. Modifications of technique are departures from the "normal" range of techniques applicable to neurotic children. There is no absolute psychoanalytic technique for use with children, but rather a set of analytic principles which have to be adapted to specific cases. Variations in technique represent appropriate specific adaptations of the basic set of analytic principles rather than deviations from standard technique.

Not all the children whose analyses require variations in technique are handicapped, delinquent, borderline, or particularly disturbed. The main guideline for the therapist in the application of modifications is his understanding of what is happening in the analysis, and an emphasis on acting appropriately rather than on applying one or another form of inherited and standard technical approach.

Lisa M. who entered treatment at three years nine months with severe fears of separating from her mother, was four years nine months old when the case was indexed:

During the first two months of treatment Lisa could not separate at all from her mother, who therefore had to remain in the treatment room. By the third month, the mother was able to sit on the landing just outside the

To Index: Describe special modifications of the treatment technique or setting and give the rationale for these changes. Comment on the child's response.

treatment room for a short period. Finally the therapist suggested that Lisa's mother should stay in the waiting room, which Lisa was able to tolerate for the most part. Subsequently, at times when Lisa refused to leave her mother, the therapist's response to this situation varied. If the specific reasons for Lisa clinging were known, the interpretation was given in the waiting room. At other times the mother was invited to come with Lisa, but most often the therapist left Lisa with her mother and told her to come up when she was ready. During the first six months of treatment, Lisa's increasing capacity to leave her mother in the waiting room paralleled her progressive understanding of her aggression toward her mother and younger siblings. The difficulties that did appear were increasingly dealt with by interpretation.

This example shows the gradual shift from management to the use of interpretation in handling special situations such as Lisa's inability to separate from her mother. The therapist may have been influenced by the fact that the reason for Lisa's referral to treatment was her clinging to her mother. Lisa's age is also important to consider in the technical handling of her clinging. The clinging was not a problem to her, especially as her mother appeared to have colluded with her, and this may have prompted the therapist to initiate very gradual steps in separating. A school-age child might well come to view the difficulty in separating as a problem of his own, since he is confronted with situations in which his peers separate easily. Lisa's behavior should not be seen as a specific response to the therapist or to the treatment situation, but rather as a very special problem, which she also brought to treatment, of separating from her mother outside the home. Indeed, Lisa gave every indication of wanting to come to treatment as long as her mother was in the room. The problem could be described another way: Lisa's problem was one in relation to her mother and not in relation to the therapist.

It may be objected that the use of an introductory period requiring management is not really analysis and does not make use of analytic technique. Certainly the first analytic task is to make contact with the child in order to gain the understanding on which to base particular interpretations. The automatic giving of interpretations without adequate evidence is pseudoanalytic. There are some therapists who would interpret, without further ado, that Lisa's aggression toward her mother was the basis of her clinging. This may be true, but it may equally be untrue: Lisa's clinging might have been based on her being aware of her mother's aggression toward her, which means it would have resulted from a need opposite to the need to defend against her own aggression toward her mother. This view is very different from the one which some therapists might take, that Lisa had displaced her anxiety in relation to the therapist onto the mother. Interpreting simply for the sake of interpreting is blind analysis; the analytic form is adhered to, but analytic understanding is not applied.

With another young child the modifications of technique described by the therapist did not involve the mother's presence. Doreen Y. began treatment at three years of age, and the indexing was done one year later:

A modification of technique was necessary because Doreen experienced some interpretations as a license to gratify wishes. Therefore when the therapist interpreted a wish, she often gave voice to the developing but feeble defense. What the therapist had in mind was that it was important that the developing defenses be reinforced. Accordingly she put things into words whenever possible. This was particularly the case when anal and aggressive matters were concerned. For example, when Doreen poured water on the floor and called the puddles "wee-wees," interpretations were cast on the side of restraint in an effort to reinforce the distance from the original wish to mess, by referring to her desire to make "pretend wee-wees." Also, alternatives were provided; for example, "You want to bite me but you can't. You can bite the pillow and talk about being angry with me."

Very young children like Doreen often act on their impulses when such wishes are spoken about; they take verbalization of their impulses as a license or prompting to act. In fact, Doreen had attained good control over bowel and bladder, but she was acutely jealous of her baby sister who obviously had no control and who she felt had replaced her in her parents' affections. It is useful to know these facts in order to understand that Doreen experienced an added regressive pull because of her sister, in addition to that experienced by any child with recently acquired bowel and bladder control. It would not have been so terrible if Doreen had really urinated on the floor. After all, wetting the floor is not the issue; the issue is, rather, what this experience would mean for Doreen. Once, earlier in her treatment, she had come to a session with a gastric upset and had slightly soiled herself. She had then become very distressed and humiliated. Analytic evidence from other children shows that a loss of sphincter control may lead to an extended period of regressive behavior outside the treatment setting as well as within it.

The second part of Doreen's example does not demonstrate a modification of technique, although the therapist suggested a displacement for Doreen's aggression, and the usual analytic technique is to verbalize the underlying wish expressed in displaced form by the patient. Therapists assume that putting wishes into words enables a child to contain his or her wishes in thought, but Doreen was not so unusual among children in her age group in reacting to interpretations in the way she did; hence it might be more useful to regard such interventions as a technique suitable for very young children, rather than as a modification of some standard technique.

The special needs of a blind child in analysis are reflected in the therapist's technique in dealing with Heather K., who was four years seven months old when treatment began, and six years five months old when the example was indexed:

With this blind child who had an uneven ego development, interpretations of her unconscious wishes often seemed to act as permissions to regress behaviorally. As treatment progressed, this problem increased. By the second year of treatment there were additional factors augmenting the strong pull toward regression. A new baby (her nephew) moved into her home, and her nursery school group had an influx of much younger children. At this point the therapist modified her technique to give Heather opportunities for more energetic and aggressive behavior in the garden. It was felt that allowing this outlet provided opportunities for displacement, in addition to the usual interpretative work. Near the end of treatment, an additional means of dealing with the still present "regressive pulls" was adopted in the form of ego-supportive activities, by extending Heather's knowledge and understanding of the world around her. The therapist took Heather on the subway, into shops, and for walks, helping her to integrate these experiences and to sort out some of the confusion a blind child experiences when confronted with these life situations. Heather derived both pleasure and gratification from such experiences, which helped her to extend the well-functioning part of her ego.

"Ego defects" as such cannot be analyzed, but these defects must be taken into account in the course of analyzing children such as Heather. In Heather's case, verbalization did not always have the desired effect. Therefore additional means had to be employed in order to help the child. The question must be asked about the function of the therapist in such a situation. Is it to act as an auxiliary ego, to allay anxiety, or to elicit material? In certain cases the child therapist may have to alternate or to combine these different functions, and it becomes spurious to ask which of these functions should be labeled analytic. There is a general difficulty in distinguishing between so-called parameters and special modifications which are necessary for the analysis. Parameters represent aids to or departures from the analytic method aimed at restoring the conditions for a normal analysis. In cases such as Heather's, technique has to be adapted and modified for the purposes of conducting the analysis. The modifications necessary in Heather's case should not be regarded as parameters, although the distinction may be purely academic and of no practical importance.

Jane G., who was thought to be autistic, began treatment at the age of seven years five months; her material was indexed when she was nine years three months old:

At the beginning of treatment Jane simply sat withdrawn, dangling a piece of string, and she avoided the therapist, who was trying to make contact with her. These first efforts were based on the offer of body contact, and, although initially it was rejected, later on in treatment it was clamored for, and Jane showed need for constant skin stimulation. She wanted to have her face and hair stroked, and she in turn wanted to touch the therapist, especially her lips. Still later in treatment, the therapist thought it was technically necessary to become more active in a variety of ways. She tried to get Jane interested in toys, in picture books, and in skipping rope together. Games involving showing and naming parts of the body were used frequently. Singing was used extensively, and the therapist "verbalized" things for Jane in the form of made-up songs.

ANNA FREUD   This is not really an example of a modification of technique. There is no formal psychoanalytic technique for autistic children so far, because we analysts do not know enough about the nature of the disturbance. We ony know that we are trying to deal with a nearly complete absence of communication. The example from Jane's treatment shows various attempts to establish contact with her, through the body, through toys, words, through singing, or through whatever bridge the therapist could find to reach the completely closed-up world of the child. This is not "technique" in the sense that it is a worked-out scheme of what to do and what not to do. If we knew how the breakdown in communication came about, we might know better how to reestablish contact, but we do not. In the neurotic child we are much clearer about the nature of the disturbance and therefore we have a basis for a treatment technique.

There may also be great difficulties in making contact with a neurotic child, though they should be distinguished from those connected with an autistic child. There are "noninterpretative" interventions with neurotic children too. A child's fear arising from his misinterpretation of reality may be dealt with by clarification or explanation. Many current neurotic anxieties in children are based on their past misinterpretations of reality.

ANNA FREUD   There are times when an analyst may explain some aspect of reality to a child, and it helps; but in a neurotic child suffering from anxiety based, for example, on an aggressive wish, or on a fear of punishment, explanation is not going to work. Some forty or fifty years ago when child analysis was not really born yet, an analyst from abroad came to visit Vienna and discussed his analytic attempts with a little boy of eight. The child was afraid of the house burning down in the night, and he could not go to sleep. The analyst said, "I took him out and I showed him that the house was built of stone, and that it couldn't burn; but it didn't help at all."

Modification of technique proved necessary in the case of Sammy R., a wildly hyperactive child who began treatment at the age of seven years two months and whose case was indexed after the first year of his analysis:

Sammy was referred because of his hyperactivity. From the beginning he could never keep still in the treatment setting, giving the impression of rushed and anxious running or clinging, hiding or seeking, falling or climbing, or some combination of these. His dominant mode of experience was a bodily one, and he was forever looking for physical means of controlling the therapist's actions and his own. For example, he spent the first week of treatment on top of the cabinet in the treatment room, or he fled outside into the garden or waiting room. All this was accentuated whenever the therapist attempted comments or interpretations. At one point Sammy requested hard wood and tools with which to make something. The therapist provided these, which were a direct gratification and also signified that she supported Sammy and his interests. The woodwork activity began in silence with particular roles assigned to the therapist, which she fulfilled. At the beginning, the therapist's attempts to speak were interrupted by Sammy's declarations that he did not want to be disturbed in his work and that he would leave if she did not shut up. Gradually he was able to tolerate the therapist's comments and to discuss the supply of wood and the meaning it had for him. The woodworking was the focus and anchor both for activity and for "verbal treatment." He could tolerate verbal interchanges by the end of the first year.

Although it is not recorded, Sammy may have had a pathological and acute fear of the strange or unknown, with an inability to tolerate dissonance of any sort. If this is the case, the fear would have caused him to be active most of the time in an attempt to find safe situations. With this child the therapist sought a means of establishing communication and took the opportunity he offered to use the woodworking for this end. It was a major achievement for him that he could sustain interest and sit for long enough to do the woodwork. Sammy could apparently do this as a consequence of his coming to feel safe in the situation because of his increased self-assurance. Thus the therapist described the woodworking as the "focus and anchor" for the more conventional treatment and during this period took on a supportive and sometimes a "subordinate" role. Her approach qualifies as a modification of technique because of the combination of the introduction of the woodwork soon after beginning treatment, the acceptance of the boy's exclusive concentration on woodwork for several months, and the therapist's long-lasting compliance with the patient's demands for minimal talk. These elements may only be quantitatively different from those which, among others, enter into the usual practice of child analysis.

In regard to the use of the couch in child analysis, older children or adolescents certainly may use the couch some time after treatment has begun, often quite late in the course of the work. In these circumstances, the technique of the transition to the couch and the effects on the analytic work are of clinical interest. Although this is not, strictly speaking, a modification of technique, a technical change is involved.

The couch was used in the treatment of Helen D., who began analysis at the age of eleven years eleven months and continued into her teens. The example is taken from two indexings, one made when she was thirteen years four months old, and the other at fifteen years:

There were special occasions in analysis when Helen used the couch. Early in treatment she asked about the couch, and the therapist gave matter-of-fact explanations of how and why teenagers and adults use the couch in analysis. Helen then used it on occasion to tell about fears of people dying, not wanting to look at the therapist at such times, nor wanting to be looked at by her. In the second year of treatment, following the analysis of her re-sistance as shown by her doing homework in the sessions, Helen's wish to use the couch more often was encouraged, while her fears about it, such as being looked at or being hypnotized, were taken up at the same time. How-ever, the therapist did not at this point interpret what she saw as the homo-sexual element in Helen's wish to be in a passive position in relation to the therapist. Helen used the couch during this period partially in expressing fears about her mother and grandmother dying and her sexual fears and cu-riosity, including thoughts about the therapist. Much later in treatment, Helen again used the couch, seeking gratification of wishes to feel like a baby, to be looked after and protected. She used it also as a vehicle of resis-tance, seeking to be protected from her anger and disappointment with her mother. Eventually she came to understand something of how she used the couch to express her homosexual wishes.

Arthur H. too used the couch. His treatment began when he was twelve years four months old; the example was indexed after three years and two months of treatment:

In the third year of treatment, following Arthur's description of his difficul-ties in discussing sexual matters when the therapist looked at him, the use of the couch was suggested as a help in talking. Considerable analytic work had already been done on Arthur's active-passive conflicts, which were dis-cussed again before he agreed to use the couch the following week. He feared being helpless and had fantasies that the therapist was a sadistic and overpowering person who could not be controlled if Arthur could not see him. Arthur was intensely anxious on first using the couch, holding himself rigidly, and giggling while associating to other situations felt to be danger-ous in which he was expected to "let go." He missed the therapist's facial expressions, which he had used as a response gauge. He imagined himself as a baby lying on the floor and also fantasied that the therapist was holding a lit cigarette as if to burn "someone" with it. The therapist interpreted that Arthur's anxiety was because he feared the therapist would harm him, a fear worsened because he felt he could no longer control the therapist by watch-ing him. Arthur agreed, and by the end of the first week on the couch, these anxieties no longer appeared. Subsequently Arthur brought sexual material more easily and with less embarrassment. Fantasies about the therapist were described more readily. The therapist became more of a transference figure vested with positive and negative qualities, contrasting with Arthur's previ-ous first image of him as an idealized object. After several months of using the couch, Arthur's transference neurosis became much clearer, and the therapist felt that the use of the couch was an important catalyst for this de-velopment.

A change of technique certainly occurs if the child is encouraged to use the couch for associating in the style of adult analysis and if the use of the couch is continued. This differs from a child's sporadic use of the couch for a variety of reasons, including those of enactment of unconscious impulses and resistance. Although there was only about one year's difference in age between Helen and Arthur, their mode of bringing material differed considerably, even before the couch was used. At the beginning of treatment, Helen often played, whereas Arthur essentially sat in the chair and talked. Helen's initial approach to the couch was exploratory and playful. With Arthur it was the therapist who made the suggestion that the couch be tried in response to Arthur's obvious difficulties in verbalizing embarrassing thoughts. There was also a difference in the technique used by the therapists in handling the issues of introducing and using the couch.

Both patients brought passive fantasies in response to the change, which is probably a general feature of the use of the couch. There was a significant difference between these two patients once their initial passive fantasies had been analyzed. Helen used the couch intermittently in a number of ways: for play, for gratification, for defense, for resistance, as well as for an aid in bringing difficult material. Arthur, however, once he had begun, used the couch consistently, and it seemed to facilitate his efforts to associate more freely. It also brought significant changes in the transference, including the development of a transference neurosis of a kind not often seen in child analysis. In fact, Arthur's treatment then took on many of the aspects of an adult analysis. There was no comparable development in regard to the use of the couch with Helen, and the same has been found to be true with other patients of a similar age.

Younger children use the couch more often in the ways that Helen did, perhaps simply because the couch is in the room and available like any other piece of furniture. Quite young children use the couch as a bed on which to enact their sexual fantasies. Helen may well have used the introductory explanations about the couch as a means of allowing her to play-act at being older or at being compliant, both of these being in the service of resistance. The crux of the difference between Helen and Arthur may be the different levels of their maturity, capacity to recognize inner conflicts, and acceptance of the use of free association as a tool in the analytic work. In addition, the two therapists had differing attitudes toward their patients' use of the couch from the outset, which must inevitably have affected the patients' response to it. For example, Helen's therapist adapted to Helen's changing use of the couch and readily worked with material she brought up in other ways. Arthur's therapist, however, viewed the couch as a talking place according to the adult model of psychoanalytic technique.

In each case presented thus far, the point can be made that the change of technique does not constitute a real modification. Either one analyzes or one does not, and the ideal technique would be geared to the child's needs at that stage of treatment. With children, the comparatively narrow confines of adult technique are inappropriate. The requirements of the analytic work may bring about substantial changes in what the therapist does or does not do. This is not the same as changing or modifying analytic technique, however. Some technique is incorrect; a therapist may simply play with a child on occasions when it would be much more appropriate, from a technical viewpoint, to interpret his anxieties, conflicts, or fantasies to him. If play therapy is conducted when psychoanalytic interventions are indicated, this is a substantial modification of analytic technique. It is quite clear, however, that many different measures and approaches can be adopted in order to further the aims of psychoanalytic treatment. Perhaps a new or unusual approach might be appropriate as long as the aims of the treatment are conceived of psychoanalytically. Formal qualification as a child psychoanalyst or as a child therapist does not indicate that the therapist has necessarily internalized the psychoanalytic approach or that she systematically applies it in her treatment of cases. This very delicate and difficult area requires further clarification. In particular, all therapists need to consider carefully the differences between modifications of technique, on the one hand, and the multiplicity of different psychoanalytical approaches to technique, on the other.

24

Extra-Analytic Contact

However much the child therapist might wish to model his treatment of children along the lines of the analysis of adults, many factors make this impossible. Even therapists who may wish to avoid contact with relatives and to limit their contacts to the child patient alone cannot completely avoid contact with the parents; nor can they avoid obtaining information such as a developmental history and a statement of the problem from sources other than the patient. In fact, one may seriously question whether it is desirable, or even possible, to conduct the analysis of a child without some degree of extra-analytic contact, with the possible exception of the treatment of certain adolescent patients.

There are variations in the extent to which a particular child's treatment is influenced by extra-analytic contacts. Such contacts cover a wide range of overlapping categories. They include contact with the child outside the treatment, contact with the parents, contact with other people, and modification of the child's environment. The therapist makes different uses of this extra-analytic material in the treatment.

Contact with child outside treatment

There are many situations in which a therapist may meet a child patient outside the treatment setting, as when visiting a child in the

To Index: Describe the nature of contact with the patient outside the treatment setting, the reasons for it, and the child's reaction. Comment on how it affects the subsequent analytic work.

hospital, attending a school function, or even visiting a child at home. Robert P. began treatment at the age of nine years eight months, and the indexing was done after the first year of treatment:

On one occasion, the therapist yielded to Robert's wish and attended a swimming gala at Robert's sports club, because it was felt that he needed this gratification in view of his being genuinely deprived at home. During the event, the therapist sat at a distance from the parents and did not communicate with them. Robert showed great joy when he saw the therapist there, but he had no opportunity to talk to her at the gala. During a subsequent session when Robert cleared his locker and wanted to see its "bottom," he indicated that he had thoughts about the therapist having seen him in his bathing trunks. After the therapist took up these thoughts, Robert promptly switched over to his "fault" in diving. Some time later he commented that the parents and therapist had been sitting separately, and he explained that the parents had reserved seats but the therapist had also had a good seat. Only many months later did he refer back to this incident and voice his suspicion that his mother and the therapist had talked with each other on that occasion. In yet another instance Robert insisted that the therapist see his painting exhibited in the local children's library. The therapist visited the exhibition on her own and discussed it with Robert after he next mentioned it.

Robert's therapist presents no convincing reasons for having attended the swimming gala. Nor is evidence presented that Robert needed the visit because he was a grossly deprived child. In the case of Frank O., however, the patient was genuinely deprived, his mother having deserted the family when Frank was three years old. Both he and his family had cast the therapist in the role of surrogate mother. Treatment began when Frank was seven years seven months and was indexed when he was eight years eight months old:

Frank had considerable difficulties in dealing with any separations, and to help him with this problem, the therapist consistently kept contact with him during breaks by means of letters, postcards, and the telephone. However, the therapist just as consistently refused extra-analytic social contacts with the child, such as going to tea, to family parties, or to school functions, although Frank and his family often urged her to do so. The refusal was based on the therapist's wish to avoid overemphasizing her role as a mother substitute, a role which sometimes interfered with the development of the transference and the analytic work.

The therapist's simply keeping in touch with Frank by letter over the holidays would not be considered extra-analytic by many therapists, but rather as an integral part of the analytic contact with a child. Most therapists would have difficulty in keeping strictly to a formal model of technique when confronted with a genuinely deprived child such as Frank. In similar situations involving deprived children many therapists cannot decide whether or not they are being too rigid or too yielding, or are having difficulties with countertransference feelings. It is important that the therapist always examine his countertransference and treat each case on its merits, rather than applying a formal technical model irrespective of the characteristics of the particular child.

A younger child, Susan S., had had many hospitalizations. Three years one month old when treatment began, the girl was six years six months of age when the example was indexed:

Susan's problem was rooted in a constitutional precocious sexuality which had occasioned numerous hospitalizations before treatment began. During treatment, Susan was hospitalized three times, twice for a tonsillectomy and once for an eye operation. The therapist prepared Susan for these hospitalizations and arranged to visit her during them. The therapist felt Susan needed the reassurance of these visits, and indeed her behavior showed that she was pleased and comforted by them. On one visit Susan demonstrated her castration anxiety with a toy the therapist brought her, and on another visit she showed good understanding of the other children's upset state at the end of visiting time.

It is not clear what particular reassurance Susan really needed. Was it a reassurance regarding the operation and related to castration anxiety, or was it reassurance regarding her fears of being abandoned by her mother or the therapist, and relating to separation anxiety, or both? The therapist's visit perhaps took care of both areas, or perhaps the analytic preparation of the child for the hospitalizations, including interpretations of anxiety related to the past as well as the present, was in itself reassuring and helped to diminish the child's anxieties. Ordinary compassion is a sufficient reason for visiting child patients in hospital, with the exception of those patients who might experience a visit as an intrusion. Naturally for the sake of the analysis one seeks to maintain contact with the child, but there may be other ways of accomplishing this besides visiting them.

ANNA FREUD   It is important for an analyst to keep to her role as an analyst. In preparing a child for a pending hospitalization and discussing his anxieties, the analyst might say, for example, "I'll look in on you once to see if this talk really helped." Then the analyst can make the visit as an analyst, coming with a "secret," something confidential, between herself and the patient which no one else need know about. Of course, it is best not to make such a visit if the analyst's motivation is to ward off her own hostile feelings or those of the child.

In general, the therapist should avoid giving the child reassurance, although the therapist may make such interventions as the verbalization of anxiety or the spelling out of reality which have the effect of reassuring the child. The therapist should provide reassurances when the child has a need for them, a need determined by the therapist by psychoanalytic assessment of the child at the time. Thus if the child is worried about the reality of an impending operation, it may be appropriate for the therapist to discuss what is actually involved in order to reduce the child's anxiety. It is very important that he pay equal attention, however, to the elucidation of the child's fantasies and thoughts about the situation.

Stephen V. demanded extra-analytic contact. He began treatment at the age of eight years and was indexed one year later:

Stephen periodically expressed a wish that the therapist should visit his home. This occurred sometimes when he longed for a closer and more extended relationship with the therapist but more usually when he wanted to show her something he talked about in his analysis, such as one of his pets or the attic door, which terrified him. Toward the end of the first year of treatment, Stephen's dog had four puppies, an event which featured prominently in the treatment and which could be utilized to elucidate his anger and rivalry with his mother, who had produced four children. Stephen desperately wanted the therapist to see the puppies and found it difficult to accept her explanations of why she did not think it would be helpful for the analytic work to visit his home. He took photographs of the puppies being suckled and brought them to his session. After the vacation he worked out a plan with his mother to bring the dogs in the car so that the therapist could see them briefly. The therapist capitulated and agreed with this arrangement, which involved a short meeting with the whole family and the dogs in the street outside. Stephen seemed satisfied that the therapist had shared this real experience with him, and his demands that she should visit his home subsequently diminished.

The therapist had previously seen Stephen's brothers and sisters in the waiting room, so that it did not seem that Stephen had gratified a wish for the therapist to meet his family. The patient had in fact made efforts to reduce such contacts to a minimum, and this matter had been taken up in the analysis as representing his wish to keep the therapist for himself and as expressing his anger with his siblings for sometimes taunting him for being "mad." Many demands made by patients for so-called extra-analytic contact seem to stem from a wish to show something to the therapist, as if talking about it did not carry the same weight as seeing it.

Contact with parents

Contacts with the parents of patients in analysis may be initiated or maintained by the therapist, by another member of a clinic team, by the parents, or by the patient. A number of different problems are involved in any contact between a child's therapist and the parents. First there is the question of whether there should be regular contact at all. Second there is the question of whose benefit is served by arranging such a contact. Is it for the child, the parent, or the therapist? There are analysts who wish not to see parents, taking the position that the analytic method is based solely on what arises during the treatment sessions. This view is incorrect, especially for younger children, because parents must be seen to be sure that they provide the continuing emotional and practical support required by the child to continue in treatment. Also, because parents themselves need to cope with changes in their child in the course of the analysis, they may need help the therapist can give. In addition to the usual ups and downs during treatment, there are more profound changes in attitudes and relationships which have to be accommodated within the family. If the family is not helped to find some means to do this, good analytic results may very often be nullified. Disturbed children frequently have disturbed parents who may need some help. On occasion a child-oriented contact with a parent leads to the parents expressing a wish for help for themselves.

A great deal of the decision whether to see a child's parents must depend on the age of the child. Some therapists prefer a colleague to

To Index: Describe arrangements for contact with the parents of the child analytic patient, including their frequency and rationale. Assess the influence of these contacts on the child's treatment.

see the parents; others prefer to see the parents themselves. In general, whoever sees the parent should exercise caution in giving interpretations to them, for to do so may be detrimental to the child's analysis.

ANNA FREUD   What the analyst does is based on the assessment of the child's disturbance and the mother's (or father's) disturbance. There is a wide range of possible arrangements, from simultaneous analysis of child and parent to having the mother within the treatment room even if only for a short time, to regular contacts, to occasional contacts only, and so on. If the child is of an age at which the environment still has an active influence on the formation of the disturbance, the need for contact with the parents is quite different from those cases in which the important disturbances are wholly internalized. In the latter case, contact with the parents may be limited to ensuring their cooperation and to keeping adverse influences on the treatment in check. Certainly there are exceptions, depending on the personality and disturbance of the parents and the personality of the child. Also, the therapist may decide to change arrangements about contact with the parents in the course of the analysis.

Lisa M. was three years nine months old when treatment began; the indexing was done one year later:

In view of Lisa's age and disturbance, which was her great difficulty in separating from her mother, it was thought necessary to see the mother weekly. The therapist felt the need both to help the mother understand the nature of Lisa's problems and to keep herself informed about daily happenings at home. Lisa's father was seen once at the beginning of treatment and on a few other occasions. Although for some months Lisa insisted on her mother's presence in the treatment room, she openly resented her mother's separate interviews with the therapist. Lisa suggested that she herself should come instead, or else her father, and she complained about being left at home alone with her father. Lisa was intensely curious about what her mother and the therapist did together and had fantasies that the therapist dressed up especially for meeting her mother.

There is a distinction between helping the mother and seeing her in order to get information about events at home. It is important for the therapist to keep informed in one way or another about daily events at home and school during treatment. With older children the analytic material itself contains information about these events, so that it is not so necessary to see the parents. There are things in a child's life which the therapist might not hear about at all unless a regular contact with the mother is available. For example, one might not hear anything from a child about a sleep disturbance which may be related to the current analytic work or to current family events or which may even be a long-standing symptom to which both child and family have adapted (of course, when such a family adaptation has been made, the parents are also unlikely to report such behavior). Regular contacts with the parents and patient provide the therapist with better opportunities to learn about such aspects. Without these opportunities, it might take a very long time before a symptom comes to the therapist's attention. With older children, as long as the therapist is in contact with the child's inner life, relatively less importance need be attached to information about the child. The need for information about events outside analysis arises particularly when there is some kind of interference with the flow of analytic material.

Lisa had been referred because of a severe separation anxiety with which her mother colluded. When a mother's pathology is involved with her child's presenting problems, the mother needs to receive some help and understanding about her child and their relationship. For these purposes the child therapist may be the best person to see the mother, in spite of the apparently negative reaction that the child may show as a consequence. In Lisa's case oedipal conflicts were brought into focus after the therapist and the mother met, but arrangements with the mother were not made specifically in order to elicit certain material or reactions from the child.

The treatment of Paul Q. began when he was three years four months old and was indexed when he was four years six months:

When treatment began, the therapist arranged to see the mother each week. The mother's ambivalence toward the child made her frequently mistake appointment times. Nevertheless she established a fairly good working relationship with the therapist, and she also telephoned if a crisis arose. The therapist adopted the approach of helping to support Mrs. Q. with the many realistic problems connected with raising her children without a husband. In addition, the therapist attempted to make links between Mrs. Q.'s own difficulties—such as her separation anxiety, sexualized aggression, and tendency to sadomasochistic interactions—and her handling of the children. There was no discernible reaction from Paul about his mother's contacts with his therapist, although he knew about them.

Paul offers a fairly typical and normal illustration of contact between therapist and mother. Giving direct advice to parents is usually useless; parents themselves usually find a workable solution to their problems once they come to see something of the underlying causes. Work with the parents should be child-oriented, that is, focused on the needs of the child rather than on the parent's own needs. The mother is not the patient and should not be treated as such. Material brought in by the mother in this context is information for the child therapist, and it can be put to various uses, such as helping the mother to gain insight into her own attitudes to the child or helping the analyst to understand the child's material better; sometimes it can even be discussed with the child.

The parents of the very young child, Greta F., were seen during the course of her treatment, which began when she was only two years and eight months old; the indexing was undertaken two years after she began therapy:

The therapist saw Greta's parents on alternate weeks, and both parents were equally involved in the child's treatment. They were seen separately at their own request. The father's underlying motive was to seek help for himself, and the interviews in fact helped him to curb his impulsive, excited behavior with his daughter. As Greta's symptoms improved, the relationship between her parents deteriorated, and her father, after one year, requested referral for analysis. He was not seen by Greta's therapist after he began his own analysis. The mother was able to use her interviews with the therapist to improve her handling of Greta based on increased understanding and insight. These contacts reduced much of her guilt for what she felt to be her early neglect of Greta, and her empathy and understanding for her daughter improved. However, when Greta's father started analysis, the mother too wanted psychotherapeutic contact, which was arranged. The therapist continued to see Greta's mother fortnightly to discuss events at home. Greta gradually came to express objections to her mother seeing the therapist, saying that she wanted her mother with her at home. Later, Greta acted as if the therapist had rejected her for being too small, in preference to the mother, thus expressing her feeling of being excluded as the therapist's oedipal partner. It is of interest that Greta showed no concern that any secrets were being revealed. The reasons for her objections to the meetings between the therapist and her mother were quite different.

Work with a parent which is not psychotherapy of the parent has limitations. The child therapist should treat a child and simultaneously work with the mother or father only so long as the parents' problems can be related to the child's difficulties. In Greta's case it was quite appropriate to refer the parents for further help with someone else when they began to focus more on their own difficulties than on the child's.

ANNA FREUD   There is a point which is not usually taken sufficiently into account by child analysts. With adult patients who have children, analysts see very clearly in analysis what a small part of the parents' personality is really involved with the child, and how great is the part that has nothing to do with the child. In working with the parents of a child in analysis, analysts are addressing themselves primarily to that area in the parents' inner life which is involved with the child. This refers to mothers and to fathers as well. It is quite wrong to think that because the child is so highly involved with the parent, the parent is equally exclusively involved with the child.

Among therapists who agree that the work with parents should be child-oriented, some prefer to see the parents themselves, whereas others prefer to have a psychiatric social worker or other trained person do that work and to keep in touch with them. The reason usually given for having a separate person see the mother is that it avoids too many transference or countertransference complications. Moreover, a new and inexperienced therapist may feel more comfortable not seeing the mother, and even a very experienced therapist may prefer this arrangement if the mother's pathology, such as rivalry with the child, clearly suggests that she needs to see a separate therapist.

With some children, the fact that the mother is being seen plays an important part in treatment, whether or not it is the therapist who sees the parent. The meaning to the child can change in different phases of the analysis. Children should know when such contacts occur, but it is a matter of clinical judgment how much detail about the interview with the parent should be conveyed to the child. Anna Freud, referring to a child she once treated who said, "I don't mind how often you see my parents so long as I don't hear about it," has pointed out that this raises the issue of whether it is right to collude with the child's denial of feelings about the contacts. Even if the therapist takes up these very feelings with the child, the therapist is not obliged to tell the child everything that has been discussed with the parents. The therapist picks and chooses, using tact and judgment. The analytic work may suffer if the therapist colludes with the parents, for example by keeping a family secret from the child. There are always difficulties involved in relation to "secrets," but it is still better for the therapist to know about the secret and to help the family deal with it, rather than to remain ignorant of the unmentioned situation. Very often a therapist can reveal a secret in the family to a child patient without any adverse effect; conversely a child may well be adversely affected by the existence of a secret he suspects and fears, but which has not been openly discussed with him.

The influence of the parents' attitude is shown in the case of Kenny K., six years three months when treatment started, indexed when Kenny was nine years three months:

Because of the parents' involvement in Kenny's symptoms of constipation and soiling, the therapist arranged to see both parents regularly. Eventually the work with the parents enabled them to give up their ignoring, denying, and apologizing for Kenny's symptoms. The parents' feelings of guilt in relation to their older, institutionalized mongoloid son played an important part in their relationship to Kenny. When the parents changed their attitudes to Kenny's symptoms, it became easier to take up his symptoms in the treatment. He became increasingly aware that his parents' changing attitudes to his soiling had something to do with their contacts with his therapist. Although he began to express mixed feelings about these meetings, as a direct result of the meetings the soiling problem came into the analysis.

The term *collusion* covers a variety of circumstances; it would be wrong to conclude that a child's conflict is perpetuated simply on the basis of parental collusion, although in some cases this may be substantially true. Naturally the parents' psychopathology is involved in the formation of the child's particular internalized conflicts, but the clarification of the parents' collusion in the present does not necessarily remove or diminish the internalized conflict itself. Nevertheless, clarification of apparent parental collusion makes the analysis of the child's conflict easier.

ANNA FREUD   The question is: what do parents do toward the maintenance of their child's symptoms or neurosis? Do they just join forces with the defenses and intensify them? Or do they join forces with and intensify the child's unconscious wishes? These are two quite different things. Intervention is much easier when the parents have joined forces with the child's defenses. Analysts find this quite often in cases of soiling or in feeding disturbances. It is not that the mother wants a soiling child or a child with food fads. Instead, the mother does not dare be confronted with the outburst of the child's anxiety.

It is sometimes difficult to tell from the child's initial behavior alone whether the mother is getting vicarious gratification or whether she is colluding with the child's denial. In work with parents one aim is to minimize the child's secondary gains from his disturbance. It is well known that when the parents derive secondary gains as well, the situation may become quite difficult to change, as in certain instances when it becomes desirable to move a child from the parental bedroom.

Helen D.'s case was indexed when she was thirteen years four months old; she had begun treatment when she was almost twelve:

Helen's mother was seen once each term from the beginning of treatment. Helen, however, often asked the therapist to tell her mother to be nicer to her and sometimes expressed her feeling that her mother needed treatment as well. She also wanted her mother to tell the therapist facts about the past. Helen's wish to have the therapist see the mother more frequently was understood as her wish that her mother should change. In addition, it was linked with Helen's feeling that her mother and therapist were omnipotent and could easily remove all her problems. Whenever mother and therapist did meet, Helen showed some anxiety about what mother had said.

Children in the early teens usually prefer that the therapist and parents do not meet, but an exception might occur when a child attempts to use the therapist as an ally in the struggle with the parents. Perhaps this was the case with Helen, who wanted the therapist to influence her mother to treat her better. It is likely that Helen's wish for her mother to tell the therapist facts about the past represented a resistance to the analytic work, as if the child were saying, "Don't ask me about my forgotten past. Ask my mother!" Alternatively, Helen's wish for her mother to be seen may have been because she wanted to shift her feelings of guilt from herself to her mother by having the mother tell about the past. Perhaps Helen was anxious after the meetings because she feared that her mother told the therapist some guilty secret.

The mother of the older adolescent girl, Tina K., who had begun treatment at the age of sixteen years five months, and whose case was indexed two years later, also was seen by the therapist:

At the beginning of treatment, arrangements were made for Tina's mother to have regular contacts with a psychiatric social worker at the clinic and for these contacts to be kept separate from Tina's treatment. During the second year of treatment, Tina's mother urgently requested a meeting with the therapist, who then discussed it with the patient. Tina agreed to the meeting. The mother presented the therapist with irrational demands that Tina be placed in a mental hospital because she could no longer tolerate the fights with her daughter at home. The consequences of this meeting turned out to be beneficial to the analysis in two ways. The therapist realized that Tina's view of her mother had some basis in reality, and Tina was surprised and relieved to find that the therapist "did not succumb to mother's charms."

Although it might be useful for the therapist of an adolescent to see the parents on occasion to compare his perceptions with the patient's view of the parents, this is frequently detrimental to the treatment alliance. The reason may lie in the fact that an aim in treating an adolescent is often to assist the patient to break the infantile ties to the parents. Tina's therapist handled the situation in a way which reinforced Tina's feeling that the therapist was an ally. A patient might have been expected to feel some distrust after such a meeting, but the meeting with the mother appears to have had the opposite effect on Tina. It convincingly confirmed to the therapist that Tina lived in a "crazy" world; undoubtedly this impression was conveyed in some way to the patient, which perhaps helped the patient to improve her awareness of reality.

Even with adults there could at times be a similar advantage to the analytic work for the therapist to interview a very disturbed spouse or other family member. In Tina's case, her mother insisted on seeing the therapist. With an adult this might occur in exceptional circumstances, for example when a husband refuses to continue to pay for treatment or when a patient requests the spouse to be seen. The analytic posture with adults is to analyze the patient, who is viewed as "big enough to take care of himself." With adolescent patients, there is some degree of variation among therapists about contact with parents. It is certainly not essential to the treatment to see parents of adolescents on a regular basis, though particular problems may make it desirable.

Information about the child patient is usually necessary at certain times in the course of *any* child's analysis. The need for information varies with age, circumstance, and phase of treatment. Analytic work is best served if only the minimum information is sought from outside, rather than the maximum. The therapist's contacts with parents also have other aims; one is to help the parents to cope with the changes brought about by the child's development and the analysis; another is to lend support to the parents' self-esteem, which is often threatened by the therapist's intrusion or involvement in their relationship to the child.

Contact with others

Contacts with headmasters, teachers, housemothers in institutions, child care workers, and others are sometimes necessary for a child's analyst. Contact outside the child's family was maintained by the therapist of Paul Q., who was three years and four months old at the beginning of treatment and whose material was indexed one year two months later:

Paul attended the clinic nursery school from the beginning of treatment. The therapist was in regular contact with the nursery school staff throughout, which provided a picture of his behavior outside the treatment setting.

This child's treatment room and the nursery school are in the same building. His nursery school notes and reports were available to his therapist, as is true for any other of the nursery school children occasionally taken into psychoanalytic treatment at this clinic. Because Paul went directly to his sessions from the nursery school, it is possible that in his mind there was a close link between the two.

To Index: Record the circumstances of any contact with persons outside the patient's family. Describe the child's reactions and attitudes to these contacts, and assess the effects on treatment.

This link would be similar to the one that a young child often feels exists between the waiting room and the treatment room: the child, believing that the therapist knows what goes on in the waiting room, feels that room to be an extension of the treatment room. For the therapist who is in daily contact with the nursery school, having so much extra information available about the child's behavior at school is a special situation and an advantage.

ANNA FREUD   This child presented two completely contrasting pictures, one in the nursery school and one to the therapist. I sometimes wondered if it was the same patient. In the nursery school he impressed everyone as a very masculine, rather aggressive, and active little boy. In treatment this side did not show at all. There his passivity and his depression were in evidence. The therapist saw only half the child, and I always wondered why the therapist did not make more use of her knowledge of his behavior in the nursery. Ideally, both sides should have appeared in treatment, but very often both sides do not appear. If an analyst has no knowledge about the child's behavior at school, for example, then she has to wait until the child brings the information. But if it is available from outside, the therapist is directly confronted with the question of why it is not available in the treatment.

Adults too may not bring whole areas of their lives and interests into the analysis for a long time, although such material is expected to come up eventually. In child analysis, there are areas which the child keeps out altogether and which may never be brought into the analytic sessions. Hence there is argument for wanting to have some knowledge of the child's behavior outside treatment. For patients of latency age onward, however, the more the therapist trusts her ability to hear the "psychic reality," the less she needs and wishes to get information about "external reality," although such data may be necessary and useful at certain times.

ANNA FREUD   With Paul, a whole, well-developed side of his personality was not brought into the treatment at all. It was not only that he was aggressive in nursery school and anxious in the treatment room. These could be linked quite easily, for example by understanding his aggressive outbursts as manifestations of his panic attacks. But in treatment he gave the impression of a regressed and ineffectual boy, while at nursery school he compared favorably in every developmental aspect with the other children. It also happens in adult analyses that the analyst does not hear much about some completely reality-oriented, efficient, and able side to the person. I remember a conversation my father had with someone who said about a patient of his, "A very nice person on the outside, really." My father answered, "Possibly. I only know him from the inside."

Contact with schools is a usual part of the diagnostic investigation, with the patient's parents' permission. In the case of Kenny K., the parents objected to the clinic's request for school reports. The boy was six years three months at the start of treatment and was indexed when he was nine years three months old:

The parents' secretiveness and denial of Kenny's problems were so extensive that the parents never told the school of his soiling symptom and requested that the clinic not contact the school. Instead the mother offered to bring school progress reports. It emerged in treatment that in fact the school did gain some knowledge of Kenny's soiling symptom following two "accidents" there.

Kenny's parents' unusual position of declining permission to contact the school was probably related to their shame about the soiling. A greater significance to the parents' secretive attitude only became apparent later with revelation of the family secret that the parents wished to keep from Kenny, namely the existence of the older mongoloid brother in an institution. Hence the important issue in this case proved not to be the parents' refusing permission to contact the school, especially as the child's disturbance did not center on the school. A patient's school should perhaps be contacted at the diagnostic stage to get an "objective" view of the child's intellectual and social functioning outside the home, which can be done without telling the school the exact reasons for treatment. Not only parents but certainly many children would like to keep the fact of treatment away from school, but if a child must come to treatment during school hours, his school's cooperation is required. No matter for what reason the school is contacted, it should only be with the parents' permission.

In the case of Betty H., a somewhat younger child, there was a different kind of parental involvement with the contacting of the school. Betty began treatment at the age of four years and three months; her case was indexed when she was five years six months of age:

There were two occasions during Betty's treatment when the therapist contacted the school at the mother's request. Soon after beginning treatment, the therapist discussed with the headmistress the possibility of delaying Betty's full-time attendance at school because of her need to come to treatment. The headmistress readily agreed, in view of Betty's immaturity and anxiety at school, in spite of her good level of achievement. A year later the therapist thought continued treatment was advisable for another term or so in order to consolidate newly acquired gains. The mother used school attendance as a welcome excuse to terminate treatment, which otherwise she would have been too guilty to do. She suggested that the therapist discuss the matter again with the headmistress, who felt that treatment was now completely unnecessary in view of the tremendous positive changes in Betty. The therapist was confronted with the difficulty of prematurely terminating without any indication from the child of her wish to do so. She told the child that her mother and headmistress had said how well she was doing at school.

Contact with the school instigated at the specific request of Betty's mother reflected the mother's fear of the headmistress and perhaps also some attempt to shift responsibility. In such circumstances the therapist is in the position of having to gain the school's support for treatment, which is needed just as some degree of parental support is needed. Even at the cost of changing schools, it should be the mother who supports the treatment by approaching the school and insisting that the school accommodate to the needs of treatment. In this case perhaps the mother's "treatment alliance" broke down, and she supported treatment only as long as it suited her to do so. She may also have been afraid of her hostility toward treatment. From other sources the therapist knew that Betty's mother's limitations in providing support for treatment might have been based on her own unconscious need for her first-born to achieve immediate academic distinction.

Contact with the school had beneficial results in the case of an older child, Tommy E., who was twelve years one month old when the case was indexed, two years and one-half after analysis began:

Tommy was anxious, withdrawn, and underachieving at school at the beginning of treatment. After two years of treatment, when his behavior at home had much improved, the mother asked the therapist to contact the school because Tommy still complained that his teachers did not like him. The therapist did visit the school after Tommy agreed. The school was understanding and welcomed the contact and the suggestion that Tommy might now respond positively to special encouragement and responsibility. Tommy later reported that he was much happier at school and was no longer afraid of his teachers.

Tommy's example might also be considered a modification of the patient's environment. In the present context what is significant is contact with the school at a particular point in Tommy's treatment, when the therapist felt that Tommy was ready for change under more favorable external conditions at school. Possibly it might have been even more beneficial for the therapist to have contacted the school at the beginning of treatment, but decisions about the timing of contact are influenced by a series of factors, among them being the nature of the child's problem. Child therapists are more accustomed to visit the patient's school if a child causes a great deal of trouble there. Withdrawn and inhibited children who do their work are usually ignored and all too easily continue to be ignored unless attention is drawn to them.

Although contact with school authorities and others has many points in common with contact with parents, contact with persons outside the family is often less emotionally charged for the child. There is a difference between obtaining extra-analytic information and bringing about an extra-analytic contact which a therapist's visit to school may entail. Moreover, there is an enormous difference between active searching by the therapist for additional extra-analytic information, on the one hand, and the use by the therapist of information which he may incidentally acquire, on the other.

Modification of the child's environment

Changes in the child's environment may be brought about by the therapist's deliberate influence or recommendation. Such changes may concern the child directly, as would a move from the parental

To Index: Describe the child's reactions to changes in his environment due to the therapist's influence as well as their effects on treatment.

bedroom or placement in boarding school, or indirectly, as when a parent is referred for analysis or psychotherapy.

Changes in his environment were made at the request of the therapist of Frank O., the latency age boy whose mother had deserted the family prior to the beginning of treatment. Frank's case was indexed when he was ten years one month old, two and one-half years after he had begun treatment:

Initially the therapist confined herself mainly to sympathetic support of the father in his difficulties in coping on his own with two school-age children after his wife's desertion. The father himself was in psychotherapy at the time. The therapist also refrained from intervening in the father's handling of Frank, except on one occasion when the treatment attendance was directly affected. In the second year of treatment, in addition to other problems, the father had back trouble, which required a plaster cast, and Frank became wildly anxious. The therapist then urged the father to get a housekeeper, which he did. This had a dramatically positive effect on every member of the family.

ANNA FREUD   This is not so different from the problem of analyzing a deprived child who does not have enough to eat and who is hungry. What does one do about it? One sees that the child is fed. Frank had an urgent need for a mothering person, and because of that, at the beginning of treatment he used the therapist, not for analytic purposes, but as a mother substitute. The right thing in such a case, in which the minimum caring requirements are not being met, is to say, "I cannot analyze your child until these basic needs are cared for." In Frank's case, the analysis really began only after the housekeeper arrived.

Edward G.'s therapist, who began his treatment when he was just over three years old and indexed his case when he was four years eleven months old, worked with the boy's mother:

The therapist's interviews with Edward's mother were used in general to help the mother with her handling of Edward, and this was done mostly by discussing the various possibilities and their likely results, without giving direct advice. On occasion the therapist did intervene more directly. For example, when the parents were considering getting divorced, Mrs. G. maintained that Edward knew nothing about the discussions and plans, and she was unwilling to talk to Edward about it. However, the child's analytic material showed clearly his partial knowledge of the situation, which made him extremely anxious, feeling that plans were being made behind his back, and fearful of what would happen to him. His behavior at that time at home was difficult, but the mother had not made any connection between his behavior and his anxiety about the possible divorce. The therapist showed Mrs. G. how much the child already knew, what he feared, and the necessity for reassurance from his mother. Mrs. G. then talked to Edward. She had been prevented from doing this by her own guilt at the thought of making him unhappy by talking to him about a painful topic. Edward's anxiety was lessened, and his behavior improved.

ANNA FREUD   What the child does in this example is a justified reaction to the mother's very clumsy handling as a consequence of her belief that if she did not tell the child about something upsetting, he would not worry about it. Since he of course guessed and worried, the question is, what is neurotic about that? After all, he should worry if his parents contemplate divorce. He did not even know with whom he would be staying or where he would be going. This is not really part of the analysis; it is an interference with the analysis, and the analyst always wants to remove any interference. The analyst's task here is similar to the situation with an adopted child who is supposed not to know that he is adopted but who guesses it. The parents are convinced that the child does not know, but the analyst recognizes that the child does know about it. One has to convince the parents to allow the child to know about it, in order to do away with the interference with the analytic work.

The modifications of the environment brought about by the therapists in the examples of Edward G. and Frank O. were aimed at removing interference which obstructed either the beginning of or the progress of the analyses. Removing the interference required a considerable period of working with the parents and involved more than giving the parents advice about handling the child. It is the experience of many therapists that attempting to give advice alone often fails to have any effect, because neither the child nor the parents are able to act on the advice and to make any sustained changes in the external situation. After some period of analysis, there may come a point when the child himself wishes to bring about a change. By this time the therapist's work with the mother may enable the mother to understand and act appropriately when the child says, for example, "I wish you wouldn't walk around without clothes on." If a child is old enough, usually into latency, he may himself actively attempt to turn away from a seductive situation, even if the mother makes it difficult for him to do so. For an adolescent, the situation is usually easier because the adolescent has much greater means at his disposal to change his environment. Thus he may remove himself from the home for a significant period of time.

Anna Freud has pointed out that there are difficulties for the analysis if a child is in a seductive situation over a period of time, perhaps acting out a sexual fantasy with a particular adult and enjoying it. While the seduction is going on, the total effect of it is directly opposed to the analytic effort. Only when a conflict can be mobilized in the child can there be something to work on, and part of the initial analytic task is to work toward establishing a conflict in the child in particular areas.

ANNA FREUD   What would most analysts expect from an adult in analysis after having analyzed with him the conflict regarding a seductive situation and acting out with a particular person? They would expect him to remove himself from the situation or to modify it. But a young child is helplessly exposed to the adult's action. The analyst intervenes only at that point where this helplessness becomes evident. The analyst helps the child to be removed from the situation. There was a case of an eleven-year-old boy who lived with an alcoholic and violent father. Whatever was analyzed while he lived there just did not help. Placement in boarding school had to be added to the analytic effort.

Child therapists must always keep in mind the fact that young children have relatively little control over their environment. Even if a child's conflicts and problems are internalized and analysis can help the child to understand his problems, he frequently cannot work out a new solution while his disturbed parents and their problems remain unchanged. For this reason therapists may find it necessary to work with the parents directly or indirectly in an effort to make the environment be as much in harmony with the analytic aims as possible.

In some other areas in which parental attitudes interact with a child's internalized problems, it is not quite so difficult to deal with the external circumstances analytically. For example, in the case of the child who externalizes a critical aspect of his superego and manipulates his parents into punishing him frequently and severely, the therapist must decide whether to intervene and attempt to stop the interaction, or whether it is preferable for him to let the situation develop in treatment and to analyze it there. Certainly the therapist should concentrate on the analytic work, but there are situations in which the therapist or someone else should attempt to influence the parents' behavior in an effort to break a vicious circle which hinders or disrupts the analysis.

In one relatively simple type of situation, modification of the environment is indicated and might even be a precondition for beginning the treatment. For example, a child may be in a school which places unfair academic demands on him, with the result that he has a significant feeling of failure and a marked lowering of self-esteem. It is not relevant to the child's problem whether or not the experience in an unsuitable school had anything to do with the origins of the problem; what is relevant is the therapist's knowledge that a change of school alone will not bring about a "cure" in the child. If the child is attending a school which is contributing significantly to his low self-esteem, however, it is doubtful whether analysis alone can successfully deal with the problem, as the school is continually reinforcing the poor self-esteem for several hours each day. Certainly the therapist should strongly support a change of schools if the academic demands imposed by his school place too great a strain on a child patient.

Although it may be possible to change schools, it is not very easy to change families. There are families which are marked by a high degree of shared psychopathology and in which the children are hardly ever considered in terms of their own needs but, instead, seem to be looked upon as extensions of the parents and as serving the parents' needs. Though not neglected in a physical or legal sense, such children are profoundly affected by the family pathology. They often come to assessment in latency showing a distortion of development, with an inability to maintain stable object relations, an absence of a feeling of safety and permanence, and often neurotic conflicts as well. Many therapists do not want to take such a child into analysis in view of the instability of the family and the uncertainty of such a family's ability to sustain a treatment alliance. If such a child is old enough, he may be able to sustain his own treatment alliance sufficiently well and might be able to make good use of treatment. A child who had a very good early period in life is more likely to respond to treatment than a child who had a very early disturbance in object relationships.

ANNA FREUD   I was once asked by some pediatricians whether analysis was indicated for a five-year-old girl who was brought up and lived with foster parents from early on. The foster parents had hoped to adopt the child. The true father suddenly appeared one day and claimed her. The child and the foster parents were terrified. The child refused to leave the house from that time on because she was afraid the father would appear from somewhere and take her "home," which for her meant away from home. She developed other symptoms, such as bed-wetting, eating difficulties, poor school performance, and was in a generally anxious state. The pediatricians asked whether, if it were legally decided that the child should go back to her biological parents, analysis could help the child over her difficulties. If I had such a case, in such circumstances, I could not forget for a moment that a wrong decision had been taken by the court and that the child's problems were the consequence of this. I would find it extremely difficult to work in such a situation. First the child is harmed, and then the therapist is asked to deal with the consequences of the harm. This would seem a deliberate act on the part of people who ought to know better and thus is much harder to accept than if it were the consequence of the pathology of the parents, who could not help themselves.

When a child's parents are killed in an accident, the child is naturally deeply distressed on the basis of the terrible reality, and often enough the child develops symptoms based on existing or reactivated neurotic conflicts. The therapist is confronted with the difficult task of helping the child with a real and current traumatic event and analyzing him at the same time.

ANNA FREUD   Child analysts should not neglect the appropriate support the child needs for the sake of his analysis. The child with a traumatic experience, such as the sudden loss of both parents, has all his previous conflicts stirred up in him; everything is in a turmoil and reaches the surface. There is plenty to analyze in the child after an experience of this kind, but this includes clarifying reality and helping the child with the consequences of the trauma itself.

Ideally the child therapist should be concerned with the whole child, including the child's environment, without neglecting the analytic task. The analytic task has to be extended to bring about modifications of aspects of the environment which appear to be interferences with the analytic work or obstacles to the analytic aim. When change cannot be achieved, some thought should be given to whether analysis is feasible for the child. It may well be that environmental limitations permit only some form of help other than analysis to be offered to the child.

Use of extra-analytic material

Information gained by the therapist from sources other than the child himself can be significant and can affect the therapist's understanding of the case. Questions involve the use to which such knowledge is put, whether and how it is communicated to the patient, and its effect on the analysis.

From the moment the therapist has extra-analytic information, whether or not she intends to use it, she may feel uncomfortable about her possession of it. In adult analysis as well as child analysis, therapists may feel uncomfortable about possessing extra-analytic information because in some way they feel that they are being untrue or dishonest in holding back information from the patient. But this situation is not so different from the possession by the therapist of the host of private speculations and conclusions about the patient which she never communicates to him. The analyst's feeling that she is in possession of something which she ought not to possess is what makes the knowledge a source of discomfort. She may also be afraid

To Index: Indicate the content and source of the information gained from others than the child, and how the knowledge gained from external sources is used by the therapist (e.g. whether the special knowledge is disclosed to the child or is taken into account in interpretations without explicitly disclosing it to the child).

that she will make a slip and reveal to the patient that she possesses such information and that, as a consequence, the patient will not trust her any more. She may worry that information from outside the analysis will distort her understanding of the material. Possession of extra-analytic material does indeed influence the therapist's understanding of what her patient brings, but this cannot be avoided by any conscious effort on the part of the therapist and need not be disastrous as long as the analyst uses as a guide her awareness of what is going on in the patient at the moment. The therapist must accept the fact that great areas of information will always remain unknown to her.

ANNA FREUD   Even with adults there are patients who exclude large areas for long periods of time or even for the whole analysis. With experience, the analyst may get a feeling that things do not quite ring true and may then ask about something which is not understood. Nowadays this kind of question is often frowned upon as an active intervention. Rather than being concerned with the problem of getting or not getting information, analysts should consider the kind of material which is likely not to be brought by the patient at all. For example, a child who is in a gratifying seductive relationship with a parent will not show it by the wish to be seduced in the transference. The reason for this is that the child's needs are quite satisfied outside the sessions. It is a different matter if the seduction occurred twenty years previously and the memory has remained and now is revived as an unfulfilled wish in the transference.

If she excludes any extra-analytic information, the therapist is consequently restricted to what the child selects for the sessions, and enormous gaps may exist. However, if information is obtained, deciding what to do with it is a different question. It can be misapplied, as in the case of an adolescent girl who had an older psychotic brother and who, in response to her therapist's remark that this must have been disturbing or frightening to her in her childhood, responded that she had never thought there was anything wrong with her brother at that time. She had grown up with her brother and his peculiarities and was used to him. Had she been in analysis at a younger age, there might have been no hint from the patient that her brother was psychotic. If the information had not been available from the mother, there would have been a danger of misjudging how the patient felt about the situation.

ANNA FREUD   The danger of misjudging is greater if one does not have such information. Had this girl been in treatment as a child and the therapist obtained this information from the mother, there would have been appropriate ways of using it. If the child had asked, "Why can he do that and why am I not supposed to?" the therapist could have used the opportunity to clarify the reality of the brother's disturbance, for example by pointing out his behavioral differences from other boys his age. Naturally this would have led to exploring the patient's fear, anger, and envy of the brother. Without this extra-analytic information, an analyst might make interpretations only on the basis of the child's penis envy and thus be out of tune with the child's psychic reality.

In many situations extra-analytic information is essential if the analysis of children is to be effective, especially for children under five years of age. Because their sense of time is not fully developed and for many other reasons, such very young children cannot be expected to bring material consistently in terms of past and present experience.

Although the therapist without any extra-analytic information may be restricted in her work, she is not much better off if she has some extra-analytic information, because she may have only a small and distorted part of the complete facts. There may well be many major items of information, however, knowledge of which would influence the conduct of the analysis markedly. The question of extra-analytic information is one of the real problems to which therapists have no satisfactory solution. To resolve it, one does the best one can in the circumstances, using one's own judgment in regard to advantages and disadvantages in each particular case. A dogmatic assertion about what is right or wrong in regard to extra-analytic information is a defensive stance on the part of any therapist who utters it.

Doreen Y., aged three at the beginning of treatment, was four years three months at the time of indexing:

The therapist saw the parents weekly and thus gained a great deal of extra-analytic information about Doreen and her milieu. The therapist knew, for example, that father and mother disagreed about ways of handling Doreen's sleeping problem, and she knew that the mother got enraged with Doreen when provoked. She also knew that mother was to have an abortion. It was decided that it was appropriate not to tell Doreen the reason for the mother's hospitalization. The therapist took this knowledge into account when making interpretations to Doreen, saying, for example, "I know that everyone at home is worried about mommy going into the hospital and that you are worried about it too." It was taken up at this particular time and was meaningful to Doreen not because of the abortion per se but because she had been very anxious about separating from her mother before the sessions and separating from the therapist after sessions.

Perhaps it would have been better to tell Doreen about her mother's proposed abortion, and it is possible that the therapist colluded with the mother in withholding information about it. But the parents did not want Doreen or anyone else in the family to know about the pregnancy and abortion, and the therapist felt that Doreen was too young to understand the specific reason for her mother's hospitalization; moreover, there was no indication in Doreen's analytic material that she had knowledge of her mother's pregnancy and wish to abort. It would have been difficult to tell with certainty that Doreen's anxiety was really based on her fear that the mother wanted to kill the baby. The external circumstances related to Doreen's anxiety—that is, the mother's impending separation from her daughter—made it appropriate for the therapist to begin interpreting her reactions to this current stress. Doreen's acute anxiety abated on her mother's return from the hospital in two days, and her anxiety about separating from her mother is best understood in the context of Doreen's murderous wishes toward her mother because of the previous birth of a younger sister, as well as her rivalry. It is important for the child therapist to sort out whether an anxiety in the child is predominantly reactive to a current external stress or is predominantly related to the analytic work. Ideally the analyst should always be aware of both aspects.

Extra-analytic material is often used to understand a resistance or what may even be a conscious withholding. A therapist is sensitive to the different ways in which a patient expresses himself and to the possible underlying meanings of what he relates, but even analytic receptivity has its limitations.

ANNA FREUD   A boy I once analyzed became especially charming at certain times and appeared to be very interested in finding out things about himself. It later came to light that this behavior followed his having stolen something and being worried about it. My first insight into what his behavior masked came not from him, not from what he brought in the session, but from outside the analysis.

Extra-analytic information was used by the therapist of Kenny K. not only in the analysis of a defense but also in a reconstruction at a later stage in the treatment. Kenny, who was six years three months at the beginning of treatment, was nine years three months old at the time of indexing:

Weekly interviews with the parents provided much developmental data and information about the current reality at home. In the first six months of analysis this information was very helpful in Kenny's coming to understand and verbalize his feelings better, since his defensive use of denial of affect was pronounced. As this defense was analyzed, his treatment alliance improved and the usefulness of current reality information diminished. In the third year of treatment, some extra-analytic information regarding a prolonged separation from the parents at eighteen months was used in a reconstruction which included a wish to touch his mother. Kenny had no conscious awareness of the early separation. Kenny's response was to bring further pertinent material, including a first reference to a transient period of excited attachment to one of his mother's petticoats.

The therapist used extra-analytic information to facilitate the analytic process, in particular the interpretation of Kenny's mood changes. It is clear that the therapist did not automatically consider these changes to be related to the transference at this early stage in treatment; rather they were understood in the context of Kenny's current relationships at home. Ideally it is the patient who tells the therapist about experiences outside which relate to his mood changes, but Kenny's general reticence and his particular defenses against acknowledging his feelings made this impossible for him. By using the information about the early separation, the therapist conveyed to Kenny that it was permissible for the child to know and feel about these events. In this sense, the use made of the extra-analytic material was an integral part of the analytic work, enabling Kenny subsequently to bring more information about himself.

It is a moot point whether the therapist is ever justified in using extra-analytic material in order to formulate a reconstruction rather than waiting for it to emerge in the transference. In Kenny's case the early traumatic experience, which was repressed, should have been manifested in the analytic material. It might be argued that it would eventually have emerged from within the child, and that it was of no technical use to try to get at it with outside information. But Kenny's therapist had waited three years before the analytic material developed to the point at which the extra-analytic information could be usefully applied.

ANNA FREUD   In treating an eight-year-old boy, I would not interpret something from the present directly in terms of the past, for example interpreting his wish to touch as a wish to fondle his mother's breast. He would probably understand me better if I were to say, "It is quite surprising to you that people reappear and are still there. You want to look at them, to hear their voices again, and to touch them to see if they are real." I might even add a general remark to the effect that this is the only way in which little children can express such feelings before they can talk. This might help the patient to understand his present experience, but this is very different indeed from reviving his past. Therefore I would not describe what happens in the analysis as a lifting of repression, because I do not think such experiences necessarily exist as organized memories. Some early feeling states may come back in the transference, and the therapist can speculate to what age they refer. But I do not think that telling a child these speculations will revive memories, though they may help in working through the affects historically associated with the early situation as well as with the present one. In Kenny's case, there is another explanation of his reaction to the reconstruction. He reacted to the therapist talking about his wish to touch his mother. This triggered off other thoughts about touching, such as his thoughts about masturbation, and then he confessed to his excitement about the petticoat.

In Kenny's case the way in which the therapist used the extra-analytic information in making a reconstruction seemed effective in that it made the interpretation more plausible and gave Kenny opportunities for distancing. The term *distancing* in this context refers to the patient's capacity to view himself as another person, perhaps to see the "baby" part of himself. The introduction of a temporal dimension is useful in bringing about distancing. If a patient can feel that an aspect of himself relates to an earlier time in his life, he may be able to tolerate it better. It is easier for a child to tolerate the idea that he was naughty as a small child than that he wants to be naughty now. The therapist should certainly make interpretations meaningful to the patient by mentioning the patient's present and preconscious concerns and anxieties, because otherwise the patient may not understand the true affective import of the interpretation.

Further technical difficulties may arise in the use of extra-analytic information. A therapist who holds fixed theoretical notions about the effects of early experience may attempt to impose his ideas on the material. Parents inevitably distort information they provide when giving a "history," for example by emphasizing the traumatic effects of a separation from them when in reality it was the departure of a nanny which had a lasting impact on the child.

In the case of Stuart L., the use of extra-analytic information seemed to be a turning point in the course of treatment. Stuart was eight years eight months old at the beginning of treatment and eleven years three months old at the time of indexing:

Stuart brought in very little material about events or feelings outside treatment, and therefore the therapist depended on information from the mother by telephone about significant happenings in his life. For example, in the third year of treatment the therapist learned from the mother that the father had experienced another mental breakdown requiring hospitalization. The therapist told Stuart she had learned about this from his mother, and subsequently Stuart began to talk with some anxiety about his father's fears and odd behavior. He also brought in feelings about his father's previous hospitalization, as well as his fear of himself being "mad" or "crazy" like his father. This opened a new phase in treatment, which was worked through over many months and led to a significant increase in the range of his potential for emotional expression.

There are children who are so frightened by reality events and also by attendant loyalty conflicts that they cannot bring the pertinent material into treatment. An eleven-year-old boy briefly mentioned that his family was intending to visit the father, who, he said, had gone abroad on a business trip. The therapist learned from the mother that the father had suffered a serious heart attack, that his life was in danger, and that the boy had been told. A girl of eight never mentioned that the mother often beat her; it was the mother herself who told the therapist.

Children often manage successfully to keep important and anxiety-laden events out of treatment. It may be helpful to confront the child with such information and to use it in the analytic work. The example of Stuart L. showed how he could not talk about his father's disturbance until the therapist gave him permission to, as it were, by introducing it herself. It was probably also important that Stuart was told that the information came from his mother. Two things acted together: first the therapist put something forbidden into words, and second the patient learned that his mother sanctioned his talking about the subject. Both Stuart's fear of disloyalty and his terror of being "mad" himself had prevented him from mentioning his main anxiety. Stuart's analysis progressed from the point of confrontation, but other children might feel impelled to defend even more against the emergence of anxiety-arousing material. Even in such cases the defenses are presumably more accessible to the analytic work after the confrontation, whereas before there may have been no sign of them, no evidence that the patient was keeping significant material away from the treatment.

Frank O.'s therapist used the extra-analytic information first to help in understanding the reasons for the child's anxiety in the session. The example was indexed when Frank was ten years one month old, after he had been in treatment two and one-half years:

Frank lived in a chaotic and motherless home and was often unable to bring any information about those day-to-day events which particularly upset him. His anxiety was manifested by episodes of hyperactivity in the sessions, which the therapist came to recognize as Frank's way of reacting to the upsetting external events. The therapist could find no way of gaining access to the content of Frank's anxieties, and although a great deal of work was done to encourage Frank to bring this information himself rather than to rely on the therapist contacting the father, it was often necessary to telephone the father during the first year of treatment to gain clues about what was upsetting Frank.

The example of Frank O. shows how easily a therapist can interpret a child's upset in terms of the past when it is in fact precipitated by real events in his current life outside treatment. Some therapists would maintain that the anxiety a patient is experiencing about something in his current life is actually only a reflection of an anxiety from his earlier childhood, and they would interpret the early anxiety directly. Thus Frank's anxiety about his father coming home two hours later than expected, having left him alone with his younger brother, would be interpreted as affecting him because of his mother's desertion when Frank was three. Such an interpretation neglects the child's current fear that he will be parentless, his fears about his own aggression, and also his age-appropriate need for a caretaker. Although the therapist need not deny the important and crucial role of past experiences for Frank, treatment should progress through his experience in the here and now, and should not neglect or bypass present difficulties and concerns. There is always the possibility of reconstructing something of the origins of the anxiety or symptom which is currently active.

Reconstructions of the past do not bring about a catharsis or abreaction in the case of children, with a massive release of emotion, as occurs in the treatment of traumatic neuroses in adults through the recovery, by means of interpretation or reconstruction, of the memory of the traumatic experience. Reconstructions of the past have other functions in child analysis, and these do not include the immediate lifting of repressions in the child. Certainly the child may benefit from the reconstruction, but at best the benefit seems to be due to his receiving a license to bring up material which he might not otherwise mention. If the child is provided with a temporal dimension for the frame of reference in which he can understand himself, something in the present may not seem to be so serious because he can now refer it back, in some way, to the past. The emphasis on current conscious and preconscious preoccupations should be strong indeed, for they serve the therapist as gates through which to enter the past of the child, especially when they take the form of present transference derivatives of the past. The dynamic importance of current pressures and conflicts, as compared to the persisting influence of the past, is particularly great for children.

Extra-analytic information should never be employed at the expense of the analytic work proper. But the therapist should not sacrifice valuable, and possibly crucial, information derived from extra-analytic sources which might greatly benefit the analysis. The therapist should avoid leaping to an interpretation as soon as he receives information from extra-analytic sources, but should think about it a great deal first, and if he does use it, he should do so tactfully, constantly assessing its pertinence to the treatment at any given moment.

25

Termination of Treatment

Relatively few analyses of children are terminated according to plan. Many are interrupted by various external circumstances, such as the patient or therapist moving away or a change of school. Some terminations are based on resistance of patient or parents, which is rationalized by the patient or the parents into a "valid" external reason. The wish to terminate may be the therapist's, the parents', the mother's in collusion with the child, or various other combinations. An important technical consideration is whether the termination comes suddenly or whether there is some advance knowledge of it.

The criteria for deciding on termination are related to the analytic aims. Termination criteria seem to fall into three groups: issues related to the analytic aim of restoring the child to the path of normal development; issues related directly to the progress of the analytic work itself, including the resolution of the transference; and the child's developmentally appropriate adaptation in his life outside the treatment setting, such as his functioning in school and at home as judged by the child, his parents, and the school. At intervals throughout the analysis the question of termination occurs to the therapist, the patient, or the patient's parents. Even though it may be dismissed immediately as an inappropriate thought, it is always there in the background. After analysis has been going on for some time, a problem of attendance at the analysis often arises, such as the

To Index: State the reasons for termination, the child's responses to the idea of termination, his reactions in the terminal phases of treatment, and the ways in which these were handled. Give the child's age on beginning and ending treatment. Distinguish between reactions to the act of termination, or a diminution in the number of sessions, and changes that occur when the idea of termination is raised, either by the patient or the therapist.

child wanting to play sports in the afternoon, or the parents wanting to move. The therapist must ask himself, "Is the child ready to stop treatment?" This means, "Can the child cope on his own, or does he show a reasonable prospect of making the transition to the next developmental phase?" There is no set of criteria which can be applied automatically, but some criteria do exist, which may aid the therapist confronted with the need to make a decision about a patient's termination.

Andy V. was two years six months at the beginning of treatment; his case was indexed when he was aged four years one month:

The decision was made by the supervising analyst and therapist that treatment should terminate, in its intensive form, after fourteen months, particularly if the child continued to show signs of readiness for nursery school. As these signs were forthcoming, termination was discussed with the mother. The mistake was made of not speaking to Andy about it immediately. When it became apparent that his mother had done so, the subject was then taken up with him. Termination was decided on because of Andy's symptomatic improvement and his firm establishment in the oedipal phase. In view of the strength of his progressive tendency, analysis was regarded as having been sufficiently successful to enable him to function well in the nursery school situation, that is, to move out of the closed family situation. When Andy went back to the aggressive lateness for sessions which had been a feature of the early stages of treatment, the therapist immediately took this up with him, and Andy confirmed that feelings about termination had provoked the delaying behavior by telling the therapist that he did not like him and asking why he could not come to play with the therapist every day. The response made by the therapist was that Andy had been coming to see him every day because there had been things which made the child unhappy, but now that he was so much happier, he did not need to see the therapist so often, but would come one day every week after the Christmas vacation. The content of termination material was very much concerned with his problem of being left and was dealt with by interpretation of the transference. Once the daily sessions stopped, Andy's interest in the analysis decreased.

Andy's was a good termination because the reason for terminating was related to the aim of treatment; namely to establish the child firmly in the appropriate developmental phase. The question can be raised whether being established in the oedipal phase is enough and whether it might not have been better still to continue the analysis in order to help the child negotiate his resolution of oedipal conflicts.

ANNA FREUD   This question is not difficult to answer. What was implied in the statement about Andy's settling in nursery school was that he was already finding some solution to his oedipal problems. The whole question makes any discussion about termination a difficult one, because usually the therapist foresees some of the dangers and difficulties of the next phase. If the aim of child analysis is to promote normal development, then the aim is fulfilled when the previously held-up development proceeds again. Otherwise an analyst would not want to terminate analysis with any child.

A question can also be raised about the wisdom of the gradualness of Andy's termination, of his being seen less frequently rather than stopping completely. Since the first mention of termination brought up a great deal of analytic material in the transference, it might have been better to have given the patient sufficient time to work through this phase completely before a final termination.

ANNA FREUD   It never seemed quite logical to me that terminating a child analysis should involve the complete separation from the analyst that it usually does for adult patients. With children there is the loss of a real object as well as the loss of the transference object, and this complicates matters. To make an absolute break from a certain date onward merely sets up another separation, and an unnecessary one. If normal progress is achieved, the child will detach himself anyway, in the course of time, just as children outgrow their nursery school teachers, their school teachers, and their friends at certain stages. The analyst can allow this detaching process to occur by reducing the frequency of visits, and often this is suggested by the child. The analyst then becomes a benign figure in the background for the child. The analyst can thereafter be visited and remembered on certain occasions, and should be available for this kind of contact.

A further question arises in regard to the frequent practice of ending treatment at the start of vacations, which was followed in Andy's case. This common practice may easily play into a denial on a child's part—and perhaps on the therapist's part also—that treatment is ending. The child may rationalize that separation from treatment is due to the vacation and thus avoid painful feelings. If analysis terminates when the child's routine remains otherwise the same, the child is unavoidably confronted with the reality of termination. It may nevertheless be convenient for the therapist to arrange for termination at vacation times, and vacations are, after all, natural breaks in the child's life. Anna Freud has pointed out that even after an agreed termination there should not be an abrupt ending of contact but a more gradual detaching process which may even be facilitated by a holiday break.

Sometimes a therapist and a child collaborate in handling a termination. It is extremely difficult to make "rules" about this subject. A latency girl was very upset about stopping and worked on the problem of termination for six months. She insisted that the tailing off be extremely gradual, and the therapist agreed. Finally a date was set for the last session, and the patient very much looked forward to another appointment with the therapist some months later, during a vacation. She failed to keep the appointment, but explained on the telephone that her bus had not come and that she wanted an appointment for the following day. She was given one, which she kept. A further appointment was arranged for the next school vacation. When the time arrived, the patient sent her mother, saying that she did not feel like coming. The therapist did not interpret this as resistance but sent a message to the child that the decision regarding appointments was entirely hers.

Katrina L. began treatment at the age of six years one month, and her case was indexed when she was eight years eight months:

After two and one-half years of treatment, there were signs that Katrina was entering latency and that the analytic process was working in some way counter to this tendency. Katrina was actually jubilant at the prospect of not having to come to treatment, though she also demonstrated her apprehension and fear that she would have to stop immediately. Although the therapist and Katrina first agreed to reduce the sessions to three times weekly, Katrina's need to remain in control of the situation showed when she missed one of these sessions and then said she wanted to come only twice a week. Following the next vacation, Katrina wanted once-weekly sessions, and seven weeks later she decided to finish her treatment. A feature of the last few months of treatment was Katrina's attempt to ensure that contact with the therapist would not be entirely lost, shown, for example, by her fantasies that the therapist would take one of her siblings into treatment.

The reason for leaving the detailed management of termination essentially in Katrina's control was to avoid having termination feel to her like a repetition of her experience of rejection when her younger siblings were born.

Katrina subsequently asked to be seen at intervals of about six or nine months over the two years after termination. She also sent her therapist cards at holidays, but gradually sent these less frequently. Her actions can be understood as Katrina's way of keeping control of her contact with the therapist for some time after the official termination. Anal characteristics played a part in the way in which Katrina controlled termination, but in many other respects features of her anal regressive psychopathology were much less in evidence. Katrina's initial jubilation and fears in regard to termination were probably related to her anticipation of loss, and she worked this problem through.

The patient Freda A.'s mother was involved in the idea of termination at the same time as the patient. Freda was six years five months old when she began treatment, and the indexing took place when she was eight years six months old:

After eighteen months of analysis, Freda's symptoms were considerably lessened, including her difficulties in coping with her death wishes, her provocativeness, her clinging to mother, and her inhibition in learning. Her original depressive affect disappeared in the first year of treatment, and by the nineteenth month Freda showed many signs of having entered latency. This improved functioning was noticeable at home and at school. Freda's mother repeatedly questioned the need for treatment because she thought Freda was well. At the same time Freda asked the therapist if treatment would end before her next birthday three months later, as she did not like missing school. The therapist finally agreed to end daily sessions at the twenty-second month of treatment. From this point Freda brought various reactions to the impending termination. She had wakeful nights and expressed fears about burglars and about a pony dying. Her sadness about leaving the therapist was expressed in her compiling a book of poetry as a remembrance of the analysis, a book which she could take home with her at the last session. She insisted that the therapist be a contributor. After the summer vacation she was seen once weekly for a further three months during which time there was every indication that she was enjoying and utilizing her newly freed time in age-appropriate ways. In the last session she complained that her eyes had tears from the light and then asked, "Will I never see you again?"

Two important external factors in Freda's life are not included in this description, although they must have played a significant part in deciding on termination. The mother had to bring Freda quite some distance for the early morning session and had to take a younger child with her on this journey almost every day. Perhaps of even greater importance was the impending departure of the therapist.

ANNA FREUD   A therapist who knows that he has to terminate an analysis because of his own departure sees the child's state in a different light from the therapist who is not under such pressure and who wants to continue the analysis until a successful conclusion is reached. Freda would have benefited either from longer treatment or from a more drawn-out termination and further contact. There is one ominous sign in the material around termination; namely, Freda's fears about the death of a pony. She had come into treatment after the death of an animal had awakened all her obsessional defenses and fears of death. The recurrence of this anxiety suggests that the same conflict was still there underneath and that it could be aroused at any moment. Treatment was not really complete.

Even if further treatment would have been desirable in this case, the fact that the therapist was leaving would have meant a transfer to another therapist. In every such case, transfer should be considered as an alternative to complete termination, and it should be decided whether the patient's condition warrants such a transfer. It is generally advisable for a patient who must terminate with one therapist to wait and only later start again with another therapist if necessary.

In the case of Helen D. the treatment was terminated because the therapist was leaving. Helen was eleven years eleven months old when she began treatment, and the indexing was carried out when she was fifteen:

Helen was told five months before termination that her therapist would be leaving. Throughout her treatment Helen persistently questioned the therapist about the date when treatment would end. This anxiety was understood as related to her fears of object loss, largely because of her fears of her own aggression. For example, even in her first session, when daily attendance was discussed, Helen said she was afraid that the therapist would dislike her if she came so often, and she suggested less frequent sessions. After two years of treatment Helen began to comment on her improvement, saying her troubles were better and she no longer cried at school. It was in the context of such comments that the therapist told Helen several months later that she was leaving. Helen's immediate response was to feel that the therapist was leaving because of her. She also expressed her wish to work harder in treatment, and she gave vent to her positive and possessive feelings toward the therapist. As the end of the analysis drew closer, Helen's resentment of the therapist's abandonment and of the fact that the therapist had other interests emerged and formed the basis of Helen's wish to see another therapist. It was possible to work through these feelings sufficiently so that termination was carried out as planned, with the proviso that further treatment could be arranged if it were to be needed later.

This situation is different from that which occurs with adolescents, who so often threaten to break off treatment. Here it was the therapist who was leaving.

ANNA FREUD   I would relate Helen's reaction less to her being an adolescent and more to the obsessional nature of her disturbance. It is typical of obsessional patients to put distance between themselves and the object, even talking about breaking off the treatment, and yet to cling tenaciously to the therapist. This is an expression of their ambivalence and the fear of their own aggression. From the beginning this was a feature of Helen's transference relationship, as when she said in effect at the first session, "If you see too much of me, you will dislike me." An analyst should really understand such a statement to mean, "If you see too much of me, you will notice my aggression, and if I see too much of you, I won't be able to keep my aggression in check."

Patients may vary a great deal in their responses to the problem of deciding when to terminate. The effect on the child of the therapist's decision to terminate is very different from the effect on the analysis of the child's wish to stop. The latter is much more frequently seen in adolescents. A child's preoccupation with stopping analysis, or even the expression of a manifest wish to stop, need not refer to a real wish to terminate but, rather, to a fear of being abandoned or rejected. Sometimes such a wish expressed by a child may really be a parental wish brought in by the child. Some patients bring many feelings about the question of termination once the subject has been raised and show the therapist that there are problems which still have to be worked on. In a significant number of cases there is a return of symptoms, or even a worsening of symptoms, as a response to impending termination. Whether this is a resistance is questionable. Perhaps in some cases it is. Freda's fear of death may have returned as a sign of her resistance to termination; it may have been a sign to the therapist that she did not feel ready for the ending of her analysis. As Anna Freud has pointed out, the return of symptoms toward the end of an analysis may have many meanings in addition to the possibility that there is more working through to be done in connection with the symptoms themselves. The return of symptoms can also mean, "I am the same at the end of treatment as at the beginning, and therefore treatment never existed." It is not always easy to differentiate between what is left to do and what is a recapitulation of the past as a reaction to termination.

In child analysis the patient's experiences of being abandoned, neglected, or separated from the mother play an important part in the child's reactions in terminating. The need to work through these responses and defenses against the loss of object is an integral part of the work of termination in child analysis. It requires working on the problem of the resolution of transference ties as well as on the tie to the real object.

Part Five

The Outcome
of Treatment

26

Aims of Treatment

To analyze is always to use a means toward an end, even though the aims of treatment might change during the course of the analysis. The question of the relation between the disappearance of symptoms and the attainment of the analytic ends is an important one, as is the whole question of the therapeutic aspect of analysis. It has often been said that the therapist should have no aim in the therapy, except to analyze.

ANNA FREUD   Analysts should distinguish between aim and method in psychoanalytic treatment. The analyst's aim is stated in terms of the patient's needs. The analyst's method is not to concentrate on these needs during the course of treatment but rather to direct attention to the analytic process itself. The analyst reaches his aim only if he concentrates on the process. It is very much like driving somewhere. Your aim is to arrive, and if instead of looking at the road, you think how nice it will be when you arrive, you will probably have an accident. Concentrating on the driving process implies steering the car. The aim and the method are different.

Aims do not necessarily change, but there are short-term aims and long-term aims. Certain acute situations, such as "school phobias" or

To Index: State the initial aims of treatment in relation to the child's psychopathology as discerned at the diagnostic stage, taking into account all other relevant circumstances. Describe more specific aims than the general one of restoring the child to the path of normal development (e.g. lessening dependency on the mother, resolving conflict over aggression). Note modification of aims as treatment progresses, with reasons. Specify limitations imposed on aims by the specific pathology of the child (e.g. ego defect, brain damage, blindness).

other intense anxiety states require a short-term therapeutic intervention. Analysis should continue when the removal of the presenting symptom is not the major aim of treatment. The therapist must
determine how to keep a child in treatment after his symptom has
disappeared.

ANNA FREUD   If a child comes into treatment because of a school
   phobia—that is, for symptomatic treatment—the analysis might
   very well end when the child returns to school, and this is not always such a bad thing. I once helped a girl with a severe school
   phobia by working with the mother. The child went through a
   very unhappy period at home because of her intense death wishes
   toward her mother. When this repressed hostility became conscious, the child returned to school. But now she became an independent and even rebellious child in contrast to her former overly
   good, passive, and compliant personality. If this had taken place
   during an analysis, the motivation for continuing treatment on the
   part of mother and child could well have disappeared with the
   child's return to school. The analyst might then have viewed this
   outcome as a resistance manifested by a flight into health. But in
   fact, inner changes had taken place which justify the view that the
   child had achieved a new way of dealing with her conflicts.

A ten-year-old boy had a school phobia which disappeared in the
first year of treatment, although his analysis continued for several
more years. His school refusal was a very small part of his general
psychopathology, which involved an overattachment to his mother,
who he feared would poison him. In this case there was a long-
standing disturbance which came to attention only because of the
school refusal symptom. It became evident, however, that the motivations of the patient and his family were not linked simply to the
school symptom but were also connected with many other disturbances.

   An instance of a limitation imposed on the analytic aims occurred
in the case of a latency girl who was suffering an acute anxiety state
for which she was referred for treatment. Kathy S. was aged ten
years two months at the beginning of treatment and eleven years
nine months old when her case was indexed:

At the beginning of treatment the main aim was to enable Kathy to move forward from the preoedipal level, to which she had regressed as a consequence of her long-standing conflict over her death wishes toward her mother. When referred, Kathy was in an acute anxiety state precipitated by a recent series of illnesses, deaths, and accidents in the household. After one year of analysis, additional aims of treatment were seen to be: a modification of her sadistic and demanding superego based on a defensive identification with her argumentative and sadomasochistic mother, and a modification of her unrealistic ideal self based on the parents' ambivalent attitudes and expectations of her. At this point in treatment it seemed that Kathy's development to date, together with the intensely ambivalent mother-child bond, would limit the degree to which these aims were likely to be achieved at present.

In addition to the general aim of restoring the child to the path of normal development, more specific aims formulated at the beginning of treatment can localize the disturbance to specific areas, such as Kathy's conflicts over her death wishes to her mother and her subsequent anal regression. But formulating more specific or intermediary aims normally requires some period of analytic work.

ANNA FREUD   Kathy's case is a good example to show the difference between aim and method, which may sometimes appear to be in opposition. For example, if the aim is to help the child make new adaptations to her conflicts over her death wishes, the method may require the recognition of these wishes. The analysis may then be perceived by the child as giving license to them, which can be a threatening and frightening experience. Also, it might be useful to distinguish between realistic and unrealistic aims of analytic treatment. Both patients and analysts often expect to achieve things which cannot be achieved by analysis. Such unrealistic expectations lead to the idea that the treatment has ended prematurely, that the analyst did not do it right or the patient did not cooperate. Perhaps analysts should pay more attention at the diagnostic stage to the limitations in aims in a particular case, taking both internal and external circumstances into account.

The example of Arthur H., an adolescent, shows how initial aims can be modified later in treatment. Arthur was twelve years four months old at the beginning of treatment and was indexed when he was aged fifteen years six months:

At the beginning of treatment Arthur was sad, depressed, lonely, and suffered from a sleep disturbance. The aim of treatment was seen to be the achievement of some measure of well-being manifestly lacking in him. Later in treatment it emerged that his functioning was severely restricted by his manifold defenses against affects and by a most intimate and ambivalent tie to his mother. The aim of helping Arthur to achieve distance from the sado-masochistic embroilments with his family was limited by the family's continual and openly expressed hostility to him and by Arthur's need to idealize the loved object.

The formulation of intermediary aims required a period of analytic work with Arthur. It is possible that at the beginning of treatment the therapist recognized neither the intensity of the family's mutual involvement in sadomasochistic interactions nor the degree to which Arthur was involved in them. Only after working with Arthur for some months did it emerge that an intermediary aim could be pursued, namely assisting him to achieve some distance from these involvements. This particular aim was probably aided by the age-appropriate adolescent move toward greater interest in the peer group and away from the family. In Arthur's treatment there did not seem to be any limitation of the aims as was seen in the treatment of Kathy S.

Psychoanalytic treatment does not mean simply "analyzing" a case. Specific aims should be taken into account by the therapist as soon as appropriate, while he still maintains the analytic posture and the analytic attitude. This requirement raises questions about the distinction between child psychoanalysis and child psychotherapy, but that distinction lies in a different area from the aims of treatment. The therapist departs from child analysis and enters the realm of psychoanalytic psychotherapy when he intentionally limits himself to specific procedures and avoids following the material into certain areas or avoids making use of any of the wide range of child psychoanalytic techniques available when such techniques are indicated. Child psychotherapy is a modification imposed by analysts or therapists on the basis of an a priori selection of techniques. The child therapist who gives only transference interpretations is practicing psychotherapy rather than psychoanalysis. Formulating relatively specific aims in regard to the particular child patient does not mean localizing the interventions or departing from the analytic procedure. Certainly the formulation of intermediary aims affects the analysis and the choice of material to be interpreted. However, many points of choice occur during an analytic session, both from the side of the patient and from the side of the therapist. There is no such thing as a blueprint for a correct analytic session, as a great deal depends on the skill and sensitivity of the child therapist.

The case of Helen S. illustrates how under certain circumstances it may be necessary to formulate limited aims. Helen was six years five months at the beginning of treatment and eight years eleven months when indexed:

Initially Helen was referred for analysis because of a learning problem. However, as the months progressed, she was found to be a very anxious and insecure child with many very early traumatic experiences, an unsympathetic, unsupportive present environment, and probably a low intellectual endowment. Consequently a reassessment of the aims of treatment was necessary. In fact, work in the first fifteen months of treatment enabled her to begin to read and to learn in school, but the success of this work was based on support, encouragement, and occasional active help with her schoolwork. While some analytic work was done, such as helping Helen to deal with her poor self-image, the treatment was a mixture of analytic and educational techniques. Realizing that boarding school would provide a safer and more secure environment, the therapist aimed at preparing Helen for such a move. This required considerable work in sorting out the confusing relationships in her aunt's family, with whom she lived.

In Helen's case there was no real change or limitation of analytic aim but, rather, a change from analytic aims to other aims.

ANNA FREUD   This case was misdiagnosed. Helen was not a suitable case for analysis but a severely deprived and traumatized child who suffered from a consequent personality distortion and who needed help, support, encouragement, and sympathy. The analytic method was not right for her, both because of the nature of her disturbance and because of her external circumstances. Analysts at the Hampstead Clinic have now had sufficient experience with children like this to know that the analytic method does not help them. They are children who have been unloved by their mothers from the beginning, who live in chaotic homes, and who are totally insecure about who cares for them. Special skills are needed to help such children, based on a psychoanalytic knowledge of developmental needs. These skills involve the proper mixture of interpretation, support, and sorting out of the confused reality. It must not be forgotten that interpretation always depends on there being an ego able to make use of it, something which is deficient in these children. Also, the disturbance is due not so much to internal conflicts as to a mixture of early neglect and damage, lost opportunities for development, unavailable permanent objects, and all sorts of adverse environmental influences.

It is difficult to supply something to a child that was missed earlier in the child's development. The therapist may help the child to make adaptations to deficits and distortions, as was done to some extent with Helen S. It might seem not really necessary for a therapist to see a child five times a week for this, when perhaps a therapeutic nursery school might also provide the needed support and encouragement unavailable elsewhere, so that development might proceed. But it is preferable to have psychoanalytic understanding and a one-to-one relationship. Ideally, the advantage of having a child therapist or analyst see a child who has suffered some deprivation is that both the analytic and the ego-supportive elements can be provided by the same person. The neurotic conflicts which are often present in such children as well can then be dealt with. Nevertheless, an analytically oriented auxiliary worker can, in many cases, provide a great deal of appropriate help, and it is not absolutely necessary that an analyst or psychoanalytically trained therapist be involved.

There is an inevitable evolution of aims during the course of analytic treatment. The beginning global aims relating to the restoration of the child to the path of normal development are crystallized at the time of recommending analysis as a method of treatment. Intermediary aims may emerge at the diagnostic stage but become clearer as the work with the child proceeds. These intermediary aims take account of the limitations imposed on the work by internal and external factors.

27

Assessment and Follow-up

Even without formal assessment of child patients at the end of treatment, much can be learned from case material, which illustrates many different elements related to termination. Because indexing or other recording of case material is usually undertaken when a child is still in treatment, there is a paucity of recorded follow-up material. Although some children do not maintain contact with their therapists, others do so over a long period of time, and their records provide information on follow-up. The issues that are related to follow-up arise mainly from the side of the therapist.

Assessment at termination

Paula W. began treatment at three years four months of age. It was terminated when she was four years seven months old, and the indexing was carried out after the conclusion of treatment:

At termination Paula was in the phallic-oedipal phase of development. She was more in control of her impulses, her object relations were less ridden by ambivalence, and her self-esteem was greater. Her general level of anxiety diminished as conflicts were resolved, and her powers of concentration and application showed improvement. These were taken as early indications of

To Index: Picture the main points of the child's personality at the end of analysis (a complete metapsychological or clinical assessment should not be attempted). Describe the phase of development reached, together with changes in ego functioning, defense organization, object relationships, areas of residual conflict, symptoms, and psychopathology. Assess how much change was brought about by the analytic work and how much change (or lack of it) can be attributed to other influences (e.g. developmental or environmental). Predict future development and adaptation, if possible.

moves toward latency. However, her conflicts over expressing anger were possibly insufficiently analyzed, shown principally by her avoiding the expression of hostility toward the therapist. She could express hostility at home. Whereas some of her father's seductive behavior and frightening angry outbursts lessened during the course of Paula's treatment, these factors remained influential in Paula's conflicts. Danger points in Paula's development were seen to be, first, a tendency to cling to the mother as a response to the mother's wish to keep her a baby, and second, a withdrawal into fantasy and perhaps the sexualization of certain situations as a result of the father's behavior.

ANNA FREUD   The problem is in providing an answer to the central question of this case, namely, the extent to which the analysis has been successful in undoing the results of the father's seductiveness and in counteracting the child's early experiences. Without saying so explicitly, the analyst is concerned with this question, implying that the tendency to sexualize is still present and that the danger of the child later repeating the parents' marital problem in her own marriage remains.

The difficulties in making predictions are enormous. For example, if treatment is terminated when the child is four and one-half and is still in the phallic-oedipal phase, the therapist cannot really predict what the child's latency will be like. Since a successful analysis is not equated with complete resolution of every conflict, it may be more useful for the therapist to formulate at the outset certain questions related to the aims of treatment and then to address herself to these questions again at termination in order to ascertain in what way a particular problem has been dealt with, and to what degree. It might be asked, for example, whether treatment would counteract the adverse effects on Paula W. of her father's seductiveness. Would treatment enable her to free herself from the adverse effects of the mother's intense involvement with her? And so on. Perhaps criteria of average expectable development should be used as a basis for assessments such as these. Even at the end of the most successful treatment, as judged by any criteria, some disturbance can be seen. Perhaps no treatment at this age could prevent the child from repeating in her own life the parents' marital pattern. After all, a child will usually be exposed to the family for many years after treatment. In fact, these questions imply an assessment of treatment as well as an assessment of the child. It may be asked how worthwhile and how effective this analysis was. Although this is not directly a question of technique, it is relevant to the evaluation of various technical approaches.

Dorothy J. was also very young, and although her analysis lasted longer than did Paula W.'s, her case presented similar problems about making predictions, especially with respect to environmental influences. Dorothy began treatment at the age of three years nine months and was indexed after she terminated treatment at the age of seven:

Dorothy's defenses at termination were seen to have been sufficiently modified to permit a considerable increase in available affect and a greater tolerance of her dependency needs and of her wishes for exclusive possession of the object. However, difficulties remained in the expression of her needs and wishes directed toward her mother. Treatment was helpful in preventing a more permanent sadomasochistic relation to her mother and in facilitating Dorothy's making the step into the oedipal phase. The environment provided only minimally appropriate objects; the father had deserted, the mother was chronically depressed and had a temporary boyfriend living in the house from time to time. Environmental factors thus constantly undermined Dorothy's efforts to make an "adequate" oedipal resolution. Moreover, identification with the mother was militated against by the mother's dramatic lack of success in functioning as a wife and mother and ultimately by her desertion of the children. Any prediction must take account of Dorothy's mode of active mastery of the environment, of her precocity rather than regression, a feature which was apparent at a very early age. It is possible that her feminine development may therefore be made difficult in regard to adopting a receptive-passive feminine position, and this could influence her object choice. Much will depend on Dorothy's ability in latency and adolescence to make use of models for feminine identification, and on the adequacy and relative permanence of available models, such as the father's second wife, with whom Dorothy is now living.

The example from Dorothy's case is highly conceptualized, although it is still possible to see past the concepts to what was actually going on. It is clear that accurate predictions of Dorothy's development will depend to a great degree on the interplay between the internal and the external events in her life. The therapist refers to this by mentioning the quality of the love objects which may be available to her. Dorothy had a significant vulnerability to depression, the reasons for which lay in the relation between Dorothy and her depressed mother and in the defensive nature of Dorothy's overly self-reliant, controlling, and cheerfully optimistic attitudes.

Predictions at termination have the problem of tending to assume the most favorable circumstances for the child in the future. There is also another difficulty. Any assessment and prediction at the end of an analysis may be affected by the fact that the therapist thought things were going well enough to agree to termination. Ideally, the therapist would like to wait a while to see how things settle down after termination before making any kind of prediction. The only valid predictions are those relating to what the therapist feels has not been sufficiently dealt with in treatment. For example, in Dorothy's case, her remaining difficulties regarding her relationship to the mother provide a basis for predicting possible difficulties in feminine sexual development, in object relations, and in her defensive structure.

Frank O. was seven years seven months old when treatment began and eleven years six months at termination. This was a relatively long analysis for a young child (three years and eleven months), and the illustration includes a chronological description of gains and achievements in treatment:

Once treatment began, Frank was easier to handle at home, and he stopped his unmanageable behavior at school, though his academic performance was poor. The analytic work of the first year of treatment enabled him to experience the rage and misery associated with the loss of his mother when he was five years old. This restored his affective contact with reality and lessened his need to withdraw into fantasy. In the second year of treatment the focus was on Frank's feelings around his mother's desertion, following her obtaining an abortion. The analysis of his jealous anger against his mother and the unborn child, together with his guilty fear of the omnipotence of his wishes, allowed him to yearn for a mother substitute and then to make a good relationship with the au pair girl. Her subsequent departure reactivated fears and fantasies associated with his mother's desertion. The analysis of this material finally led to Frank's being able to accept the au pair girl's departure with appropriate sadness and regret, and to express the wish for a successor to replace her without fear of disloyalty. During this year he was better able to tolerate separation, he wrote letters to the therapist during vacations, and his schoolwork improved somewhat. Still vegetarian, like the rest of his family, he now ate reasonably well and with pleasure. In the third year, signs of latency development appeared. Though he had no satisfactory mother substitute at home and was still very attached to the therapist, the transference lost its initial intensity and Frank could foresee and acknowledge a time when he would no longer come for treatment. Attempts to use the therapist as a need-satisfying object were by now only occasional and were chiefly in the service of resistance. His object relationships matured; for example, he maintained a more realistic appraisal of his absent mother, and he made his first real and lasting friendship with another boy. In the fourth year, Frank's hostile anal wishes were worked on, leading to a freeing of aggression and a sudden and marked improvement in his schoolwork, securing for him a prize for the best schoolwork of the year and also a place at grammar school. He was able to separate from his family successfully when he went to a school camp for a vacation, and he could maintain quite good relationships with his brother and father, while hoping some day his father might marry again. At termination Frank was functioning appropriately at a latency level with regard to sublimations, object relationships, and defense organization, in contrast to the conflicts, the need-satisfying level of object relationships, and primitive defenses evident at the beginning of treatment. In particular, defenses such as projection, clinging, denial, and withdrawal into fantasy had largely been supplanted by more appropriate use of passive-into-active, repression, and sublimation. Significant areas of incomplete analytic work included Frank's relationship to his father. Although he became aware of and tolerated hostile feelings to his father, Frank was not able to work through these feelings as thoroughly as he did in regard to his absent mother, probably because he still needed his father so much. Another such area was on the oral level, where there was evidence of a fixation point associated with early and only partially satisfied dependency needs. The analysis was hampered in this area because of the continuing real deprivation at home throughout the treatment. In view of Frank's remarkable ego achievements, it is unlikely that these would be impaired in any future difficulty. However, he might experience difficulties in the sphere of object relationships, for example in the capacity to retain a loved object or to deal with depression at the loss of such an object.

Anna Freud has contributed significant follow-up information to this example. Some time after treatment was ended, Frank's father remarried, and the stepmother became pregnant and had a baby. Frank was very hopeful about having a good relationship with his stepmother but was disappointed in this. She was idealized at first but did not live up to his expectations. Then, two and one-half years later, when he ran into difficulties in adolescence, he had a striking breakdown in ego functioning. He could no longer get on at school, losing all pleasure in learning and work. These difficulties were all the more striking in view of the amount of analysis that he had undergone. Anna Freud commented that someone who had suffered traumatic object loss to the extent that Frank had would always be more susceptible than others to the experience of loss in the future. However, she thought it was incorrect to expect that his ego achievements would remain unaffected, and events proved her right. The prediction should have been made that there would always be a strong link between his ego achievements and the gratification derived from his object relationships.

Arthur H., an adolescent, was assessed at termination and the analytic work was traced through changes in defensive functioning, instinctual development, object relationships, and changes in his internal conflicts. Arthur began treatment at the age of twelve years four months and was indexed after termination when he was fifteen years six months old:

Arthur began treatment as a sad and highly defended child with little pleasure in life. At termination he appeared as an active and introspective adolescent who derived pleasure from a variety of interests and relationships. The changes in the manifest picture are related to changes brought about by the analytic work. When treatment began, Arthur was almost totally occupied in warding off drive gratifications and a wide range of affective experiences. He utilized extreme forms of externalization and projection, phobic avoidance, and a great deal of intellectualization and rationalization. The analytic work enabled him to feel less frightened, so he could permit himself less distance from his impulses, which were previously severely inhibited. He more readily allowed a variety of affective reactions and came to recognize spontaneously some of his own defensive maneuvers to avoid anxiety. A tendency to displace and to project remained, but the persecutory element in his defensive processes had virtually disappeared. Arthur's intense phallic conflicts had led to major regressive moves in his development, particularly in his object relationships. He had developed an extreme inhibition of phallic exhibitionism. With much analytic work in the areas of his castration anxiety and his masturbation conflict, Arthur gradually became more assertive and masculine in behavior and appearance, and he began to relate to girls in an age-appropriate manner. A major change in Arthur's object relationships came with the analysis of his relation to his mother, with whom he had a most intimate, ambivalent, and sadomasochistic tie. Initially, aspects of this relationship were displaced onto other objects, particularly sadomasochistic involvements, enactments of passive-active conflicts, and identification with the aggressive woman with the aim of warding off an anticipated castrating attack. The analysis of his rage and his disappointment in the depressed mother of his early childhood permitted Arthur to accept people as they were, instead of tending to idealize them. However, he retained a tendency to externalize his high standards, so that people often failed and disappointed him. Perhaps related to this was a persistent fear of close and intimate relationships. This had been worked through to some extent in the transference. It was felt that, with termination, he might be freer in this area. Arthur's harshly severe superego constantly condemned any experience of pleasure or gratification. He persistently saw himself as "not good enough," and he suffered intense guilt, self-condemnation, and painful depression. The analytic work focused on the introjection of highly ambivalent images of his mother and of the sadomasochistic relationship with her, which had resulted in his becoming both victim and attacker in relation to himself. This work allowed Arthur to see himself in a more positive light, to experience pleasure, and to reduce the masochistic satisfaction from attacks on himself. However, it seemed that Arthur would always have very high standards of achievement and behavior and that he would remain prone to feeling guilty for failures to live up to his ideals.

This example highlights the difficulty of making predictions. In Arthur's case it would appear that the therapist justifiably restricted himself to delineating areas of change and to describing those aspects of Arthur's pathology relevant to his future development and about which there was some doubt. For example, although the therapist described how Arthur's fear of close relationships was a feature of the transference and had been a focus of the analysis, some doubt was conveyed regarding the degree of freedom he had in fact attained. The therapist may have felt that the continuation of the patient-therapist relationship itself contributed significantly to the perpetuation of Arthur's difficulties in this area, and that only termination would offer him the opportunity to find a resolution. These seem to be the kinds of question that could be posed at termination without having to go into the issue of prognosis. This is as true of adult as of child analysis. Arthur was an adolescent and, therefore, for developmental reasons had greater opportunities to break with past modes of relating and to make new inner and outer adaptations.

In general the example of Arthur gives a good account, in a number of dimensions of the analysis, of the areas where changes occurred and where limits were reached. Of concern here is not child analytic technique as such but, rather, the therapist's view of what the treatment had or had not achieved.

Follow-up after termination

Relatively few cases of children who have been analyzed provide follow-up material. It might be useful for research to make contact

---

To Index: Cite information about the patient obtained from later contacts with the child, with his parents, or others (e.g. school or child-care officers). Note whether these contacts are maintained, entered into, or resumed after the termination. Record the dates of contact, together with the reasons for the contact and relevant details about the child's functioning after analysis.

with every patient's family at least one year after the patient's termination, perhaps by approaching the patient or his parents, inviting
contact if there were any problems as well as requesting information
about the situation of the child. But such an approach does not consider the needs of the patient. Instead the most useful follow-ups are
those initiated by the former patients or their parents themselves.
Another difficulty has to do with who sees the child and the parents.
Although a "real" picture of the child might not be obtained if someone other than the original therapist is involved, that therapist might
get too subjective a picture to be useful if he assesses the case himself.

In assessing cases where contact is made or maintained after termination, the therapist should clarify whose wish initiated the contact, and how it was made. The child's ex-therapist should examine
very carefully his own motives in regard to maintaining contact.
Some therapists continue contact by sending birthday and Christmas
cards after termination. This might become a permanent commitment, for to stop sending them might be felt as a rejection. Other
therapists may send two or three such cards and, if the child does not
respond, then stop. But some parents or children might feel a sense
of obligation to reply. Experience suggests there is some selection by
therapists of which children are sent cards, since no one appears to
make it a practice to send cards to all ex-patients.

One aspect of contact with the child after analysis is related to
what use the child has made of the therapist. The therapist is a real
person for the child patient, which does not contradict the fact that
the therapist has also made contact with the child in a very different
way from anyone else. Later in the child's life, the remembered
therapist will be a special person or a special friend. The degree to
which this image contains elements of therapist-as-therapist seems
related to a number of factors. These include the age of the child at
the time (thus young latency children might well exclude "analytic"
functions from this image), the nature of the transference relationship at termination, and the degree to which the child has taken over
the analyzing functions of the therapist.

ANNA FREUD   Analytic technique never included the idea that it is
    wrong to break off relationships completely after treatment has

ended. As far as the relationship is based on transference, it should end, but insofar as it is a real relationship, the child should be left to outgrow it gradually.

Adults occasionally come back for more treatment after the formal termination of analysis, especially if a crisis has occurred.

ANNA FREUD   Children find it more difficult to return to analysis than adults, apparently being kept away by some sort of resistance. The question remains as to why a great deal of resistance may have been kept secret during the analysis and only afterward come to light. Often a child's treatment is terminated with the idea that, in a year or two, the child will come back if more therapy is needed, but this hardly ever happens.

What happens after termination is also related to the manner and extent to which the transference developed in the child's analysis and the degree to which it was resolved. A man aged twenty-three, who underwent analysis as a child, beginning when he was seven, still maintains occasional contact with his therapist, particularly by telephone. He turns to his therapist as to someone who is strong and who will protect him from a stronger female, such as his mother. In this instance, although there is an element of an unresolved treatment relationship, the patient continues to use the contact to help him to cope with real difficulties.

The reasons for which a former child analytic patient makes or maintains contact vary greatly. Another ex-patient, still a child, telephones her therapist every term. At termination there were still problems about loss which had not been worked through, and the contact afterward consisted simply of talking about apparently trifling things. For the patient it seemed simply to be a reassurance that her therapist was still there. It is possible that the child was still trying to deal with her loss. Other children make contact only if and when they have a problem or crisis, as in the case of the young man of twenty-three. If a child has used a therapist to a significant degree as a real object during treatment, then he will tend to use the therapist after termination for the solution of reality problems. Yet if the therapist was used primarily in the analysis to deal with internal problems, the child may be more reluctant to open up these problems again. With very young children, much of the experience of treatment may be repressed as part of the infantile amnesia.

Another kind of problem about making contact appears to exist when the treatment has been stopped by the parents after symptomatic improvement. The child may have conflicts about the treatment being stopped at that time, and the therapist's making or maintaining contact in such a situation may occasionally increase the difficulty between the child and his parents and may even put the child into a conflict of loyalties.

When the therapist is contacted after the analysis, it is important that she first try to assess the reason for which the contact is being made. For example, if the parents have sent the child because they are anxious about one or another aspect of the child's behavior, the therapist has first to try to find out what the basis is for their worries. Her approach will be very different from the one she would take if the child had contacted her of his own accord and had brought his own difficulties or conflicts to the therapist who had helped him in the past. In all these situations, there is a problem of the degree to which the therapist shows herself as a "real person" and to what extent she maintains an analytic stance with the patient. Whatever the ostensible reason for a particular visit, its meaning for the child may not always become clear in one interview alone, and it may be necessary for the therapist to see him several times, although not necessarily daily.

The therapist's attitude toward a particular termination often influences the way later contact with the former patient is viewed and handled. Some therapists, anxious and concerned about a patient's ability to get along on his own, offer their home telephone number and make an appointment for some later time. This seems to be the case particularly when the patient's wish to terminate appeared to be premature and was only reluctantly agreed to by the therapist. Contrasting with this attitude on the therapist's part is another which indicates that the therapist is not easily accessible anymore to the patient. He may show this inadvertently by expressing irritation; or he may suggest directly that the patient should by now be able to cope on his own. All sorts of countertransference problems get drawn into this situation.

Sometimes the parents of an ex-patient contact the therapist, as did the mother of Freda A., who had begun analysis at the age of six years five months, and whose treatment terminated when she was eight years six months old:

One month after termination, Freda's mother phoned the therapist to report that Freda had had an accident and to ask if it needed special handling. Freda's father had dropped her at the crossroads on the way to school, telling her to cross over at the proper crossing. She did so but was hit by a car. The first thing Freda then asked was whether it had been her fault. Freda was unhurt but needed to be hospitalized for a few days for observation. The mother described the child as being depressed and not wanting to stay in the hospital. But after the first day she made friends with the other children, liked the nurses, and was in good spirits. She expressed anger at the driver of the car which hit her. The therapist felt that the telephone call was for the mother's own reassurance, especially when she said that she always had fears that something like this might happen to Freda. When the mother inquired if she should tell Freda about the phone call, the therapist suggested that it was not necessary. The reason for this was to draw Freda as little as possible into the parents' anxieties and conflicts, which seem to have been stimulated by the accident.

ANNA FREUD   There is not much in the mother's call to be dubious about. In fact, considering Freda's previous problems about death, accidents, and guilty feelings over death wishes, I would be quite concerned if the mother had not notified the therapist after the accident and asked questions about her daughter. It seems entirely appropriate to have reassured the mother, and it would also have been appropriate to suggest that she tell the child she could come to see the therapist when she was out of the hospital to tell the therapist all about the accident.

Apparently Freda's therapist thought that the mother made the phone call simply because of her own problem, that the mother's death wishes toward her daughter had been stirred up by the accident, and therefore the mother was seeking reassurance for this reason. From this point of view it seems that the mother, who had had no analysis, made the contact because it was she who needed help. However, because the therapist was Freda's therapist rather than the mother's, her predominant concern should have been with Freda. It might have been better if she had suggested to the mother that she should tell Freda to contact her.

It is important for certain children to have continued contact with the therapist in one form or another, though certainly in a very different form from the analytic setting. Some children can be left to avail themselves of the therapist if a crisis arises. For others, complete and final termination by the child himself should be considered appropriate and not pathological.

ANNA FREUD   Child analysts do not really know at present which cases need variations from and additions to the analytic technique that has been developed. Analysts are interested in the limits within which analysis is the method of choice, and this is the question we have pursued over the years at the Hampstead Clinic. Full internalization of conflict does not occur for many years, and the child may need help with the environment. Therefore, in child analysis, assistance from both sides is needed—internal help for the method of coping, but external help for undue pressures on the child. These questions are especially relevant for the youngest age group, for whom the conflicts with the environment are so important.

Case Index

Andy V., 84, 134, 146, 190, 242–243
Arthur H., 96–97, 172–173, 206, 207–208, 253–254, 262–263
Betty H., 223–224
Calvin S., 180–181
Charles Z., 148, 196
Doreen Y., 201–202, 233–234
Dorothy J., 58, 61, 111–112, 147, 259, 260
Douglas O., 179–180
Edward G., 102, 155–156, 226–227
Esther L., 55, 81, 90–91, 157
Frank O., 110, 120, 136, 139–140, 143, 161, 170–171, 176–177, 178, 210–211, 226, 227, 238–239, 260–262
Freda A., 71–72, 245–246, 267
Greta F., 138–139, 143, 184–185, 216–217
Heather K., 202–203
Helen D., 12–13, 109–110, 132, 205–206, 207–208, 219–220, 246–247
Helen S., 64–65, 255–256
Ilse T., 86, 166–167, 191
Ingrid C., 119
Jane G., 203
Jerry N., 22, 76, 142, 146, 160–161, 194–195
Karen C., 88, 89
Kathy S., 252–253, 254

Katrina L., 11–12, 75, 94–95, 141–142, 143, 161–162, 167–168, 244–245
Kenny K., 31–32, 35–36, 112, 154–155, 218, 223, 235–236
Kevin C., 99–100
Lisa M., 102, 199–201, 214, 215
Lydia S., 167
Mary G., 130
Michael B., 28–29, 81, 85–86, 148, 165–166
Norma Y., 134–135
Oliver U., 37
Paula W., 257–258, 259
Paul Q., 128–129, 189, 195, 215–216, 221, 222
Quentin J., 23, 49, 66
Richard B., 128
Robert P., 166, 210
Ronald I., 132–133, 145
Sammy R., 204–205
Stephen V., 212
Stuart L., 237–238
Susan S., 12, 159, 160, 175–176, 178, 211
Tammy L., 40–42
Tina K., 100–101, 140–141, 143, 148–149, 220
Tommy E., 129–130, 135–136, 160, 224–225
Victor C., 119–120

General Index

Abreaction, 186; Anna Freud on, 70, 121. *See also* Repression

Acting out, 84, 137–143; as mode of expression, 117, 139; distinguished from enactment, 137–140; and idea of resistance, 142; defined, 142–143; for defensive reasons, 143; as free expression, 189. *See also* Dramatization; Enactment; Play; Role playing

Addiction, 27. *See also* Object relationships

Adolescents: and resistance to treatment, 15, 87, 247; and parents, 15, 50, 93, 97, 220, 254; and treatment alliance, 50, 54–55, 56; and mistrust, 56; regression fears of, 86–87, 96, 97–98, 100; intellectualization by, 91; and transference/transference neurosis, 93, 101, 103; and displacement from, 100; externalization of problems by, 106; and ideals, 107; verbalization by, 119–120; techniques with, 199; therapist's contact with parents of, 220–221; and modification of environment, 228; and termination of treatment, 247, 263

Age, of child: and treatment value, 10; and transference, 82, 103; and explanations, 161; and adult restrictions, 190; and physical contact and gratification, 192; therapist's contact with parents of, 213–215; and follow-up, 264. *See also* Latency development

Aggression: as reaction to interpretation, 75; to self-observation, 124; as mode of expression, 134, 189,

190–191; acceptance of, 173. *See also* Gross bodily discharge; Restrictions

Aichhorn, August, 52

Aims of treatment, 251–256; Anna Freud on, 251–256 *passim*; distinguished from method, 251, 253; modification of, 253–256

Alexander, Franz, 70, 96, 111

Ambivalence: of parents, 9, 55; splits in, 102–103, 107; of obsessional patients, 247

Amnesia, infantile, 15, 266. *See also* Repression

Anal-sadistic symptoms, 88, 89, 172

Analyst. *See* Therapist

Anxiety: and wish for help, 45; as reaction to interpretation, 58, 75, 76, 142, 162; as focus of interpretation, 63, 179, 234, 239; relief of, 64, 134, 173–174, 189, 212; defense against, 73, 179–180, 196, 238; about therapist, 79, 98; working through, 184–185, 186. *See also* Guilt; Separation anxiety; Verbalization

Assessment at termination, 257–263; Anna Freud on, 258, 264–265, 267, 268

Attachment, to treatment: and therapist, 26, 31, 79, 89, 94–95, 98, 103, 153; and treatment alliance, 47, 53. *See also* Object relationships; Transference; Treatment alliance

Attendance, 7–16; and number of sessions, 7–8, 16, 70, 243, 244–245, 246, 256; Anna Freud on, 7–16 *passim*; daily treatment, trend away from,

7–9; therapist's attitude toward, 8, 9, 14, 15; irregularity in, 9–10, 11–12, 13, 79, 144, 160, 188; and guilt feelings, 49, 97; commitment to, 49. *See also* Resistance; Termination

Autistic children, 203–204; Anna Freud on, 21, 203

Auxiliary ego. *See* Ego

Behavior: and transference improvement, 94; flight into health, 94, 252; change of, 145; interpretation of, 187; free expression, 189; sexual, 190–191. *See also* Acting out; Aggression; Homosexuality; Interpretation; Regression; Restrictions; Modes of expression

Blindness: and auxiliary ego, 108; and speech, 119; techniques for, 199, 202–203

Bolland, John, 3, 84

Bringing in material, 117–136. *See also* Nonverbal expression; Verbalization

British Psycho-Analytical Society, 1

Bulletin of the Hampstead Clinic, The, 1

Change of setting, 35–42; Anna Freud on, 36, 38, 39, 40; child's reaction to, 36–37, 40; preparation for, 37–38; therapist's reaction to, 40; and transference, 90. *See also* Modification of environment

Change of therapist, 26–34; Anna Freud on, 27, 28, 29–30, 32; as abandonment, 28–29, 32, 247, 248; wish for, 30–31, 247; three types of, 32; vs. termination, 32–33, 246; preparation for, 33–34. *See also* Termination

Character: resistances, 58; transference, 79, 80. *See also* Resistance; Transference

Clarification: of interpretation, 158–163, 204; of parental collusion, 218. *See also* Collusion; Interpretations

Collusion: of parents with patient, 160, 219, 241; of therapist with patient, 197, 218; with defense, 165, 168–169; with parents, 218, 219, 234. *See also* Treatment alliance

Coming and going, 144–149; bringing in material, 117; Anna Freud on, 144,

147; change of behavior in, 145; role playing in, 147–148. *See also* Attendance; Extra-analytic contact

Communication, 121, 125; and treatability of child, 118; and opposition to, 126; and autism, 203. *See also* Modes of expression

Confrontation, 163. *See also* Extra-analytic contact

Conscience, 49. *See also* Guilt

Contact, 36, 206. *See also* Extra-analytic contact; Physical contact

Corrective emotional experience, 70, 96; regression in, 110; deprivation and, 111; vs. correcting experience, 113

Couch: fear of, 16; vs. visual contact, 36, 206; purpose of, 188; effect of, 205–208

Countertransference. *See* Transference

Defense: and displacement, 37, 84, 165; and resistance, 59; insight as, 72; against anxiety, 73, 179–180, 196, 238; play as, 75, 125, 136; habitual mode of, 81; apparent transference as, 87; against transference, 91; choice of, 91; intellectualization as, 91; and homosexual transference, 101; externalization as, 109; nonverbal expression as, 123, 124, 129–131; acting out as, 143; interpretation of, 158–159; collusion with, 165, 168–169; against speech, 168

Deprivation, emotional, 106; and corrective experience, 111; and countertransference, 211; dealing with, 255–256. *See also* Reality events

Displacement: vs. transference, 27, 82, 84, 102; defensive, 37, 84, 165; play as indicator of, 75, 123; as extension of the present, 82–83, 85, 89; regression and, 85; adolescents and, 100; interpretation aids and, 164, 165. *See also* Externalization; Spillover phenomenon

Distancing, 21; as aid to interpretation, 166, 167; from direct sexual expression, 176; as term, 236–237; obsessionality and, 247

Dramatization, 117, 121, 131, 132; danger of, 167. *See also* Acting out; Enactment; Interpretation; Play; Role playing

Drawing, and painting: as mode of expression, 117, 121, 131; as aid to interpretation, 167. *See also* Nonverbal expression

Ego, the: and treatment alliance, 46–47, 54; verbalization and, 68, 121–122; insight and, 68, 69, 70, 71; and auxiliary ego, 107, 108, 162, 202. *See also* Superego

Ego defect, 105, 202, 256

Ego-dystonic experiences, 73

Ego resistance, 59. *See also* Resistance

Ego-syntonic disturbances, 72

Emotional deprivation. *See* Deprivation

Enactment: in symbolic play, 31, 120, 129; and verbalization, 120, 122–123, 138, 191; awareness of, 124; through motor means, 137; and acting out, 137–140; restrictions on, 188, 189; and couch, 207. *See also* Acting out; Gross bodily discharge; Physical contact and gratification; Play; Role playing

Environment. *See* Change of Setting; Modification of environment

Expectations. *See* Fantasies

Expression. *See* Modes of expression

Externalization: self-observation and, 68, 69, 71; transference as, 78, 79; and regression, 96; facility for, 97; adolescents' wish for, 106; interpretation of, 106, 109; as defense, 109; interpretation aids and, 164, 165; and therapist intervention, 229. *See also* Displacement

External world. *See* Reality events

Extra-analytic contact, 209–240; with child, 149, 209–213; use of, 160, 231–240; and working through, 184; Anna Freud on, 211–212, 214, 217, 219, 222–223, 226–236 *passim*; with parents, 213–221, 223–231, 235, 237–238; with others, 221–225; and change of environment, 225–231; after termination, 264–268. *See also* Coming and going; Parents

Fantasies, and expectations, 62–66, 156; about interruptions, 20, 22, 23, 24–25; about change of therapist, 28–30, 31, 34; and transference, 40–42, 62, 63, 64, 66, 86, 100–102, 141; verbalization of, 51–52, 62–63, 66, 118, 119, 121; interpretation of, 62, 66; Anna Freud on, 63–65 *passim*; and treatment alliance, 63, 64, 65; and resistance, 63–64; of external change, 64, 105–106, 138–139; and transference neurosis, 99; nonverbal expression of, 121, 123, 128; and toys, 126–127. *See also* Sexual fantasies; Play; Reality events

Fixation, 88–89. *See also* Regression

Folkart, Lydia, 12

Follow-up after termination, 263–268; Anna Freud on, 258, 264–265, 267, 268

Franctionated analysis, 21. *See also* Interruptions

Free association: resistance to, 57, 58, 59; role of, 57, 155, 190; play as equivalent of, 124–125, 127

Free expression, 189. *See also* Behavior

Freud, Anna, 40, 88, 105, 162, 165, 190, 195, 228, 261; founds Hampstead Clinic, 1; influence of, 2; on indexed material, 3. *See also* individual entries

Freud, Sigmund, 82, 109

Frustration, 197. *See also* Physical contact

Gratification. *See* Physical contact

Gross bodily discharge, 117, 123, 131, 134, 137, 171. *See also* Aggression; Enactment; Modes of expression; Restrictions

Guilt, feelings of: in change of therapist, 31; about missed sessions, 49, 97; and resistance, 60; awareness of, 73; aggressive response to, 75, 124, 133–134, 189; vs. fear of punishment, 109; reduction of, 135; interpretation of, 177. *See also* Anxiety

Hampstead Child-Therapy Clinic, 24, 52, 70, 127, 255; founding of, 1; orientation of, 2

Hampstead Psychoanalytic Index, The, 3, 84

Homosexuality: and couch, 16, 206; and treatment compliance, 16, 55; anxiety about, 79, 179; and transference, 101; acting out of, 141. *See also* Sexualization

Hyperactivity, 204–205, 238

Hysterical conversion, 140. *See also* Acting out

Id elements: in treatment alliance, 53

Identification, with therapist: and treatment alliance, 47; as insight, 72; and transference, 107, 109, 112

Indexing procedures, 2–3, 257; scheduling and attendance, 7; interruptions, 17; change of therapist, 26; change of setting, 35; treatment alliance, 45; resistance, 57; fantasies and expectations, 62; insight and self-observation, 67; reaction to interpretations, 74; transference, 78, 79, 82, 87, 92, 99; other uses of the therapist, 105; bringing in material, 117, 118, 123, 131, 133; acting out, 137; coming and going, 144; introducing treatment, 153; clarification and confrontation, 158; aids to interpretation, 164; significant interpretations, 170; selection and timing, 175; working through, 182; restrictions, 187; physical contact and gratification, 192; modifications of technique, 199; extra-analytic contact, 209, 213, 221, 225, 231; termination of treatment, 241; aims of treatment, 251; assessment and follow-up, 257, 263

Infantile amnesia, 15, 266. *See also* Repression

Insight, and self-observation, 67–73; *Krankheitseinsicht*, 46, 72; and treatment alliance, 46–47; capacity for, 50; Anna Freud on, 68–72 *passim*; development of, 68, 69, 73, 184; and working through, 70, 184; as defense, 72; interpretation and, 76; verbalization and, 119, 124; aggressive reaction to, 124. *See also* Working through

Intellectualization, 91

International Journal of Psycho-Analysis, 2

Interpretation, aids to, 76, 164–169; Anna Freud on, 165, 168–169; choice of, 167; overuse of, 168; use of song as, 173. *See also* Play; Role playing; Toys

Interpretations: rejection of, 12, 74–77, 176, 180; student analysts and, 38; Anna Freud on, 38, 74–76, 113, 129, 158–159, 165, 168–169, 171, 177, 178, 182–183; of sexual fantasies, 40–41, 128–129, 138–140, 142, 146, 175–176, 179, 235, 236; anxiety about, 58, 75, 76, 142, 162; in advance, 60–61; of fantasies, 62, 66; avoidance of, 62, 63; focus of, 63, 179, 234, 239; aggressive reaction to, 75; acceptance of, 75, 76, 77, 179; phrasing of, 76; and somatic symptoms, 76; guides for, 99; of externalization, 106, 109; vs. experience, 113; of play, 129; during play, 132; acting-out reaction to, 142; clarification of, 158–163, 204; of content and defense, 158–159; significant, 170–174; selection and timing of, 175–181; and working through, 182–186; of early trauma, 185–186, 239; insufficiency of, 187; of aggressive activity, 191; inadequate evidence for, 200; as license, 201, 202; and noninterpretative interventions, 203, 204; extra-analytic information and, 233, 235–240; distancing in, 236–237; of current anxiety, 239; and ego, 255–256. *See also* Working through

Interruptions, 17–25; Anna Freud on, 17–22 *passim*, 24–25; and resistance, 18, 19; reaction to, 19–20, 90, 210; by therapist, 20–21; fantasies about, 20, 22, 23, 24–25; change of therapist and, 33; and transference, 90

Intervention: verbal, 120, 122–123, 135, 158, 190, 212; and acting out, 142; noninterpretative, 203, 204; Anna Freud on, 203, 204, 219, 226, 228, 229, 232; and parents, 219, 226, 228, 229. *See also* Extra-analytic contact; Interpretations

Introducing treatment, 153–157, 200; Anna Freud on, 155, 157

Katan, Anny, 68

Kennedy, Hansi, 1

Krankheitseinsicht. See Insight

Latency, 252, 264; infantile amnesia
and, 15; interruption of treatment
and, 21, 23–24, 244; contrasted to
prelatency and adolescence, 86–87;
and mode of expression, 131,
135–136, 139–140, 141; and sexual
material, 176; prediction of, 258. *See
also* Age

Mistrust: basic, 56; as habitual mode,
80; extra-analytic information and,
232. *See also* Object relationships;
Treatment alliance
Model, Elizabeth, 12
Modes of expression, 117–149; derivative forms, 121, 138; Anna Freud on,
121–122, 124–127 *passim*, 129, 130,
134, 137–138, 144, 147; and aids to
interpretation, 167; nonverbal,
187–188. *See also* Acting out; Aggression; Bringing in material; Coming
and going; Nonverbal expression;
Play; Restrictions; Verbalization
Modes of relating. *See* Relating
Modification of environment, 225–231;
patient's demand for, 64, 105–106,
138–139. *See also* Change of setting;
Change of therapist; Extra-analytic
contact; Fantasies; Reality events
Modification of technique, 199–208;
Anna Freud on, 203, 204
Motor activity. *See* Enactment; Gross
bodily discharge; Modes of
expression

Narcissism, 59, 72
Neurotic conflicts, 186, 199, 229, 230,
256; Anna Freud on, 203, 204. *See also*
Transference
Nonverbal expression, 123–131; and
treatability, 117–118; and fantasy,
121, 123, 128; as defense, 123, 124,
129–131; Anna Freud on, 124–130
passim, 134; of negative feelings, 131;
and verbalization, 131–133; changes
in, 132, 133–136; as regression, 133,
189; restrictions on, 135, 187–191; by
therapist, 162; need for, 187–188. *See
also* Modes of expression
Number of sessions. *See* Attendance

Object relationships: and reaction to interruption or termination, 20, 22, 23,
243; and change of therapist, 27–28,
34; adult addicts and, 27; transference as, 50, 78, 161; and mistrust, 56,
80, 232; and extension, 82–83, 85, 89;
in transference neurosis, 92–93, 95;
interpretation of, 106, 109, 128; instability of, 229–230. *See also* Attachment; Displacement; Externalization;
Relating; Therapist; Transference;
Treatment alliance
Obsessionality, 179; about attendance,
13; and change of setting, 35; and
need for help, 46; ego split and, 68;
and precocity, 68–69; and self-observation, 71; and analytic hour, 95, 162;
and verbalization, 120; at termination, 246; and distancing, 247

Painting. *See* Drawing
Parents: ambivalence of, 9, 55; resistance of, 9, 10–11, 12, 51, 160, 224,
241; adolescents and, 15, 50, 93, 97,
220, 254; and change of therapist vs.
termination, 32; child's relationship
with, 42, 47, 81, 96, 98–99, 100, 102,
154, 217, 253, 254, 259, 262–263; and
treatment alliance, 51, 224, 229;
therapist's role with, 99, 105, 162,
211–212, 213–221, 266–267; collusion
with child, 160, 219, 241; intrusions
of, 178; pressure from commitment,
188; contact with therapist, 213–221,
223–231, 235, 237–238; collusion with
therapist, 218, 219, 234; and contact
with school, 223–225; distortions of,
237. *See also* Extra-analytic contact
Parent-syntonic symptoms, 11
Payment: and nonpayment as resistance, 9, 220; attitudes toward, 10,
188
Permissiveness, 83–84, 99, 133, 188,
191; and regression, 94–96, 135, 162.
See also Restrictions
Physical contact, and gratification, 137,
192–198; and fantasies, 64, 138–139;
insight into, 72–73; and therapist, 96,
113–114, 193–194; pitfalls of, 123; as
reassurance, 162; restriction and,
189–191, 193; Anna Freud on, 194,

197, 232; demands for, 196–197, 232; license for, 201, 202; as modification of technique, 203, 204–205. *See also* Extra-analytic contact

Play: symbolic, 31, 120, 123, 129, 177, 178; materials for, 39, 126, 128–129, 171, 188, 198; as defense, 75, 125, 136; as mode of expression, 117, 123, 132, 189; as intermediate stage, 121; as free association, 124–125, 127; Anna Freud on, 124–129 *passim*; as resistance, 125, 136; and verbalization, 131–132; therapist's role in, 131–132; as interpretation aid, 164; as working through, 184–185; as modification of technique, 208. *See also* Acting out; Toys

Projection, 78, 96, 109. *See also* Externalization

Psychoanalysis: distinguished from psychotherapy, 7, 22, 254; essence of, 57; modifications of, 199–208

Psychoanalytic Study of the Child, The, 12

Psychotherapy: distinguished from psychoanalysis, 7, 22, 254; as modification of environment, 226

Rationalization: by therapist, 8; by child, 71

Reality: explanation of, 158, 159, 212; misinterpretation of, 204; psychic vs. external, 222

Reality events: distinguished from resistance, 12, 19, 177; importance of, 14, 36; reaction to, 42, 82, 230–231, 237–238; and transference, 82; and interpretation, 177–178; intrusions of, 178; and traumatic experience, 185–186, 239. *See also* Change of setting; Change of therapist; Deprivation; Extra-analytic contact; Intervention; Modification of environment; Spillover phenomenon

Reassurance: about treatment, 156, 157, 161–162; reality as, 158, 159, 212; nonverbal, 162; as adjunct to interpretation, 163; in extra-analytic contact, 211, 212; following termination, 265, 267. *See also* Physical contact

Receptionist, function of, 194

Reconstruction of past, 186, 239. *See also* Abreaction; Repression

Regression: in current relationships, 83, 85; in ubiquitous behavior, 86; fear of, 86–87, 96, 97–98, 100; fixation point in, 88–89; permitted, 94–96, 135, 162; to ideal mother-child relationship, 96; and corrective experience, 110; nonverbal expression as, 133, 189; of fantasies, 147; anal-sadistic, 172; need for, 188–189, 198; sphincter control and, 201. *See also* Permissiveness

Reich, Wilhelm, 40

Rejection. *See* Separation anxiety

Relating, habitual modes of: transference of, 79–82, 88; vs. regression, 86; adolescent break with, 263

Relationships. *See* Object relationships; Parents; Spillover phenomenon; Therapist; Transference; Treatment alliance

Repression, 15, 59, 239, 266

Resistance, 57–61, 153; by parents, 9, 10–11, 12, 51, 160, 224, 241; in absenteeism and tardiness, 9–10, 11–12, 14, 160; and interpretations, 12, 74–77, 176, 180; and reality, 12, 19, 177; vs. treatment alliance, 12, 45, 49, 180–181; by adolescents, 15, 87, 247; holiday as, 18, 19; and "Monday crust," 21–22; change of therapist as, 30–31; transference as, 48, 100; vs. basic unwillingness, 55–56, 57; Anna Freud on, 57–60 *passim*, 21; to free association, 57, 58, 59; and character resistances, 58; defense and, 59; and ego resistance, 59; anticipation of, 60–61; interpretation of, 63; and fantasies or expectations, 63–64; play as, 125, 136; acting out as, 142; demand for information as, 161; role playing as, 167; aids to interpretation and, 167, 168; vs. working through, 185; extra-analytic information and, 234; to termination, 247–248; "flight into health" as, 252; after termination, 265. *See also* Interpretations; Interruptions

Restrictions, 187–191; relaxation of, 135; Anna Freud on, 187–188, 189; distinguished from discipline, 190; and gratification, 193. *See also* Permissiveness

Role playing: and role reversal, 86, 112, 140, 147–148; fantasy in, 123; in coming and going, 147; as interpretation aid, 164, 166–167. *See also* Acting out; Dramatization; Identification; Interpretation

Sadomasochism: in child-therapist relationship, 49, 154; insight and, 71; tendency toward, 79; persistence of, 89; in child-parent struggle, 98, 154, 253, 254, 259, 262–263
Sandler, Joseph, 2, 3, 84
Scheduling. *See* Attendance
Schools: therapist's contact with, 223–225; change of, 229; phobia of, 251–252. *See also* Extra-analytic contact; Modification of environment
Sealing up, 21, 24, 147
Self-observation. *See* Insight
Separation anxiety: and interruption of treatment, 19, 22, 23–24; and change of therapist, 28–29, 32, 247, 248; and termination, 247–248. *See also* Interruptions
Sexual fantasies, 148, 160, 258; transference of, 40–41, 86, 100–102, 141; interpretation of, 40–41, 128–129, 138–140, 142, 146, 175–176, 179, 235, 236; source of, 66; and couch, 206, 207; and change of environment, 228. *See also* Fantasies; Play; Reality events
Sexuality: distancing from, 176; expression of, 190–191. *See also* Fantasies; Homosexuality
Somatic manifestations, 128; as reaction to interpretations, 76; distinguished from acting out, 140
Song, 173, 203
Spillover phenomenon, 83, 84, 85, 87, 89, 102, 141, 142–143
Split: in patient, 52–53, 68; in ambivalence, 102–103, 107
Sterba, Richard, 68
Story-telling: as interpretation aid, 76, 164, 166, 167–168. *See also* Interpretation; Modes of expression
Sublimation, 21
Superego: in treatment alliance, 46, 47, 49, 50; as conscience, 49; and insight, 70; modifications in, 107; therapist as, 162; externalization of, 229

Symbolic material. *See* Play
Symptoms: parent-syntonic, 11; relief of, 54; somatic, 76, 128, 140; anal-sadistic, 88, 89, 172; hysterical conversion, 140; return of, 246, 247–248; disappearance of, 251–252

Technique. *See* Modifications of technique
Tegelsee Sanitorium (Berlin), 27
Termination, 241–248; vs. change of therapist, 32–33, 246; child's wish for, 33, 241, 247; premature, 224, 266; criteria for, 241–243; Anna Freud on, 243, 244, 246, 247; gradual, 243, 244; therapist on, 246, 266; and return of symptoms, 246, 247–248; adolescents and, 247, 263; as abandonment, 247, 248; resistance to, 247–248; assessment at, 257–263; follow-up after, 263–268. *See also* Attendance; Change of therapist
Therapist: on attendance, 8, 9, 14, 15; cancelling sessions by, 20–21; attachment to, 26, 31, 79, 89, 94–95, 98, 103, 153; student as, 31–32, 38; humanity of, 38; on change of setting, 40; personal preoccupations of, 41; identification with, 47, 72, 107, 109, 112; countertransference by, 50, 154, 197, 211, 217, 266; contribution of, 50, 51–52, 54, 56, 220; patient's relationship to, 82–83, 85, 89, 103–104; as provider of gratification, 96, 113–114, 193–194; other uses of, 97, 105–114; role of, 99, 105, 162, 211–212, 213–221, 266–267; Anna Freud on, 106–113 *passim*; as auxiliary ego, 107, 108; as need satisfaction, 110–111; in play, 131–132, 205; intervention by, 142, 204, 219, 226, 228, 229, 232, 252; outside of session, 149, 209–213; use of extra-analytic information, 160, 231–240; and working through, 183; division of functions of, 194; collusion with patient, 197, 218; different functions of, 202–203; collusion with parents, 218, 219, 234; at termination, 246–247, 266; special skills of, 255–256. *See also* Attachment; Change of therapist; Collusion; Displacement; Extra-analytic contact;

Intervention; Modifications of technique; Object relationships; Physical contact; Spillover phenomenon; Transference; Treatment alliance

Thomas, Ruth, 12

Tone of voice. *See* Verbalization

Toys: role of, 188; changes in, 36; Anna Freud on, 39, 126–127, 194; as gratification of need, 64, 194, 195; in interpretation, 164, 168; taking home, 194–196. *See also* Play

Transference, 78–104; negative, 13, 29, 48; and clinic, 27; vs. natural response, 40; fantasies in, 40–42, 62, 63, 64, 66, 86, 100–102, 141; distinguished from treatment alliance, 45, 47–48, 49; positive, 47, 56; and countertransference, 50, 154, 197, 211, 217, 266; defined, 78, 82; four types of, 78–99; of habitual modes of relating, 79–82, 88; character transference, 79, 80; Anna Freud on, 80, 85, 89–95 *passim*, 101, 103; and transference neurosis, 80, 87, 92–99, 206, 207; of current relationships, 82–87; reality events and, 82; age and, 82, 103; of past experiences, 87–91, 92; defense against, 91; and transference improvement, 94; changes in, 99–104; defensive or homosexual, 101; distinguished from crush, 101; resolution of, 103, 241, 248, 265; vs. real relationship, 103–104; vs. identification, 107, 109, 112; and real relationship, 108; acting out in, 138, 141–142, 143; and transference derivatives, 138, 239; interference with, 161; and demands for gratification, 196–197, 232

Traumatic experience, 185–186, 239. *See also* Reality events

Treatability, 118

Treatment: introduction of, 153–157, 200; aims of, 251–256. *See also* Attendance; Payment; Resistance; Termination

Treatment alliance, 45–56, 153; vs. resistance, 12, 45, 49, 180–181; vs. treatment compliance, 16, 55; in change of therapist, 26, 34; in change of setting, 37; Anna Freud on, 45–55 *passim*; distinguished from transference, 45, 47–48, 49; insight and, 46–47; instinctual and noninstinctual, 47; trust in, 48, 56; conscience in, 49; therapist's contribution to, 50, 51–52, 54, 56, 220; adolescents and, 50, 54–55, 56; with parents, 51, 224, 229; negative, 51; definitions of, 53; id elements in, 53; fantasy and, 63, 64, 65; sustainment of, 229. *See also* Attachment; Collusion

"Treatment Situation and Technique" (manual), 3

Trust. *See* Mistrust

Unpunctuality. *See* Attendance

Verbalization: of threats, 12; of fantasies and expectations, 51–52, 62–63, 66, 118, 119, 121; role of, in early childhood, 68, 129; as mode of expression, 117–123; and self-observation, 119, 124; by adolescent, 119–120; as intervention, 120, 122–123, 135, 158, 190, 212; Anna Freud on, 121–122; and tone of voice, 122, 131; refusal of, as defense, 123, 124, 129–131; and written material, 131; and nonverbal expression, 131–136; and enactments, 138, 191; as license to act, 201–202

Working through, 182–186; and fractionated analysis, 21; and change of therapist, 29, 31, 34; and insight, 70, 184; and significant interpretations, 170, 172; Anna Freud on, 182–186 *passim*; vs. resistance, 185; and termination, 245, 248

Writing, 131. *See also* Verbalization